Ignore the Awkward!
How The Cholesterol Myths Are Kept Alive

Uffe Ravnskov

Let's be clear: the work of science has nothing whatever to do with consensus. Consensus is the business of politics. Science, on the contrary, requires only one investigator who happens to be right, which means that he or she has results that are verifiable by reference to the real world. In science consensus is irrelevant. What is relevant is reproducible results. The greatest scientists in history are great precisely because they broke with the consensus. There is no such thing as consensus science. If it's consensus, it isn't science. If it's science, it isn't consensus. Period.

Michael Crichton

This book is intended solely for informational and educational purposes. Please consult your doctor if you have any questions about your health. Because the proponents of the cholesterol campaign have misled most doctors, it may also be a good idea for him or her to read this book.

ISBN 1453759409
Copyright © 2010 Uffe Ravnskov
Cover Photo: Jan Nordén

Contents

Introduction

Now they're planning the crime of the century
Well what will it be?
Read all about their schemes and adventuring
Yes it's well worth a fee
So roll up and see
And they rape the universe
How they've gone from bad to worse
Who are these men of lust, greed, and glory?
Rip off the masks and let's see.
But that's not right - oh not, what's the story?
There's you and there's me
That can't be right

Hodgson, Roger, Davies, Rick (Supertramp)

A fad idea

Are you worried about your high cholesterol? Do you avoid butter, cheese and cream because you are afraid of dying from a heart attack? Do you take a cholesterol lowering drug? If so, you are a victim of the cholesterol campaign, the greatest medical scandal in modern times. Even worse, you may suffer from bad memory, muscle weakness, pain in your legs, sexual impotency or cancer, not because you are getting old, but because of the harmful effects from your cholesterol treatment.

Don't you believe me? Neither does your doctor because all the experts have said that cholesterol reduction is harmless.

Unfortunately they are wrong. Not only have the pharmaceutical companies and their paid researchers succeeded in presenting the cholesterol reducing drugs as a gift from heaven. The very idea that saturated fat and high cholesterol are deleterious to health is created out of thin air. In spite of that it has been accepted uncritically across the globe.

The hypothesis that is used as the argument for the cholesterol campaign has three paragraphs. First, the concentration of cholesterol in the blood goes up, if we eat too much saturated fat.

Second, when cholesterol is too high, our arteries are converted from smooth canals to rough-walled and narrowed tubes. Thirdly, because of the irregular artery wall a blood clot may be created causing a myocardial infarction or a stroke. Let us take a first, short look at them.

Saturated fat isn't bad

That saturated fat is harmful to human health runs counter to common sense. Fat is composed of various types of fatty acids and fatty acids are molecular chains of various lengths, mainly composed of carbon and hydrogen atoms. Some fatty acids lack hydrogen atoms and therefore they have one or more double bonds between the carbon atoms. They are named monounsaturated with one double bond and polyunsaturated, if they have more than one. Small amounts of mono and polyunsaturated fatty acids are necessary for normal cell function. We produce them ourselves except for a few of the polyunsaturated ones, which we need to get from our food.

Saturated fatty acids are stable molecules because they are saturated with atoms of hydrogen. One of the main constituents of our cell walls is saturated fat. We produce saturated fat ourselves to build new cells and the excess is deposited in our fat cells for later use. Saturated fat is the dominant type of fat in milk, the fluid that is able to nourish the growing baby for a long time after birth, on its own.

Do you really believe that humans are designed to produce a toxic molecule that will eventually kill us? Could the dominant fat in mother's milk be poisonous to the baby? It is simply a masterpiece of deceit to convince a whole world that too much saturated fat in our food should cause a deadly disease.

High cholesterol is good

When I heard about the cholesterol hypothesis for the first time I had just left the University of Copenhagen with an MD. The paper that raised my interest came from Framingham, a small town near Boston, where a research team had studied a large number of its citizens for some years. What they discovered was that the concentration of cholesterol in the blood of those who suffered a heart attack during the observation time had been a little higher when they entered the program. The directors had concluded that high cholesterol was the very cause of myocardial infarction.

My biochemical knowledge was still intact then and I knew that cholesterol was one of the most important molecules in our body.

It is impossible to build cell walls and nerve fibres without cholesterol. We produce other important molecules, for instance the sex and stress hormones, by changing the structure of the cholesterol molecule a little. With a little help from the sun our skin cells use the same method to produce vitamin D. Cholesterol is also of vital importance for the brain. We cannot think clearly without it. Not only is cholesterol used by the brain cells and all nerve fibres as an important building material; the chemical processes necessary for the creation of nerve impulses are also dependent on its presence. It is therefore no surprise that the brain has the highest concentration of cholesterol in our body. The importance of cholesterol is apparent from the fact that the richest source of cholesterol in our food is the egg, because much cholesterol is necessary to produce a healthy, living, warmblooded creature. Cholesterol is so important that all cells are able to produce it by themselves. In fact, every day we produce three to five times more cholesterol than we eat. If we eat too little in our diet, the production goes up; if we gorge on animal foods, it goes down. This is why it is so difficult to reduce and control blood cholesterol with diet. When you have read this book you will even realise that high cholesterol is good; the higher the better.

The idea that a little extra cholesterol in the blood should result in a deadly disease seemed to me just as silly as to claim that yellow fingers cause lung cancer, or that burning houses are set on fire by the fire brigade. I didn't pay much attention to the Framingham report, because I thought that such foolish ideas would soon be disproved by more intelligent scientists. Sadly, I was wrong.

Why I have written this book
Many people who have read my previous books have probably realized that I am a truthful person, but some readers may still wish to question me. Doesn't he know that the cholesterol campaign is led by the world's best experts? Surely, it is Ravnskov who has misunderstood the issue. Hasn't he just cherry-picked the results that are seemingly contradictory? How could it be possible to seduce a whole world of scientists?

Judge for yourself. My aim with this book is to show how white has been turned into black by ignoring any conflicting observations; by twisting and exaggerating trivial findings; by citing studies with opposing results in a way to make them look supportive; and by ignoring or scorning the work of critical scientists.

Those who have not read my previous books possibly may not quite understand the width of these misleading processes.

I have therefore included some of the most obvious contradictions to the cholesterol hypothesis, shortened and simplified.

The first part of this book deals with the studies, which have been used most often as supporting evidence by the supporters of the cholesterol campaign. In the second part, I demonstrate how they have succeeded in misguiding a whole world.

The final part of my book is about what I believe to be the actual cause of atherosclerosis and cardiovascular disease, based upon the best available scientific research. I have developed that idea together with my colleague and friend, Kilmer McCully. It was he who discovered that children born with excessive amounts of homocysteine die early because of severe atherosclerosis. I have already presented this idea in my previous book 'Fat and Cholesterol Are GOOD for You!', but because it demands some biological knowledge to fully understand it, I have tried to explain it again in another more simple way.

If you find that what I have written seems hard to believe, please consult the sources given at the end of each chapter. It is easy to obtain the documents to which I have referred. Perform an advanced Google search using the phrase "Pubmed single citation matcher". Put the name of the medical journal in the field named 'Journal', write the year of publication in the field named 'Date', the next number in the reference is the 'Volume' and the last one is the 'First Page'. You need not write the name of the authors. In most cases only the summary is available. If you want to read the whole paper, send a request to the author, whose email address may be given after the summary. If it is not, then order the paper from your nearest university library. By doing this systematically, as I have done, you will not only discover the truth for yourselves, you will also learn more about cholesterol and the heart than most doctors.

I have tried to use language that is understood by most people. Readers who want to have more details and more of the references to the scientific literature, may find them in my previous book.

The Myths

CHAPTER 1
The Animal Argument

And so castles made of sand,
melts into the sea eventually

Jimi Hendrix

The idea that a faulty diet may raise the concentration of cholesterol in the blood and lead on to atherosclerosis, first saw the light of day one hundred years ago, when Russian researchers fed rabbits with cholesterol and various types of fat dissolved in corn oil.

I have often wondered how they persuaded the animals to eat something that is completely different from their usual vegetarian food. Probably, the fluid was injected through a catheter which was put down into the stomach. In any event, the rabbits' cholesterol values increased to more than twice as high as ever noted in human beings. I assume that the cause was not only the strange food, but also the stressful situation because in human beings, mental stress is able to raise cholesterol values considerably in a short time.

After some time, the structure of their arteries had changed and they looked as if they were demonstrating early human atherosclerosis. The cholesterol wasn't localized to the arteries only; every organ took it up just as a sponge would soak up water. Thus, a process similar to atherosclerosis starts in the arteries of rabbits if they are fed a diet that is completely different from their usual one. Mice born with abnormally high cholesterol levels develop similar changes, but other animals, for instance rats and baboons, do not react in this way.

How do we know whether human beings metabolise fat and cholesterol like a rabbit or a baboon? Has any researcher asked that question? To my knowledge the answer is no. The reason is of course that nobody knows. It is a crucial question because if we are more like baboons, which I think we are, these experiments cannot tell us anything about human atherosclerosis.

Interesting information comes from studies of wild animals.[1]

Atherosclerosis is more unusual and much milder than seen in human beings, possibly because animals that are not one hundred percent fit may not survive for a long time in an environment inhabited by various beasts of prey. The latter do not become atherosclerotic, however, even though they live entirely on animal food. Atherosclerosis is seen occasionally in vegetarian animals, but most often in birds, probably because their blood pressure is higher than in land animals. It is not due to their food because seed and grain-eating pigeons, for example, and fish-eating penguins are just as atherosclerotic as the birds of prey.

Surprisingly, it is not this naturally occurring atherosclerosis, which has caught the interest. In any scientist with an open mind, many relevant questions should arise. If vascular changes, similar to human atherosclerosis, are found in some wild animals but not in others, why do they occur in the vegetarian but not in the meat-eating animals? Why have scientists studied the vascular changes created by force-feeding laboratory animals only and ignored the spontaneous atherosclerosis?

Obviously, before they start their experiments, they have already concluded that it is dietary fat and cholesterol that cause atherosclerosis and coronary heart disease. Instead of studying natural atherosclerosis, they induce vascular changes in the animals by cholesterol-feeding and call it atherosclerosis. Furthermore, it is not atherosclerosis that we want to avoid; it is its alleged consequences, such as myocardial infarction and stroke. However, although thousands of researchers have studied fat-fed animals, none of them has succeeded in producing a heart attack or another cardiovascular disease by this way.

There are a few exceptions, but this is no proof that the food was the cause, because both atherosclerosis and coronary heart disease can be seen in zoo animals fed with their natural food. To prove that the unnatural food is causal, two groups of laboratory animals should be studied, with one group given the fat food and the other group given its natural food.

Why do the researchers continue with these experiments? Why do very few ask themselves, why atherosclerotic animals never suffer from a heart attack? The answer may be that it isn't atherosclerosis itself that causes heart disease, but something else. I believe that I know the nature of this unknown factor and how it may lead to the production of a clogged artery. In the final chapter I shall tell you more.

Fat fruit flies

Recently professor Carl S. Thummel and his co-workers at Utah University reported their revolutionary experiments on fruit flies.

They have discovered that fruit flies become fat and their cholesterol may go up for the same reason as in human beings – a high-fat diet. According to Thummel we have here a simple way to study the interplay between cholesterol and atherosclerosis because fruit flies are much cheaper than mice and rabbits. In addition, we will get a quick answer because the average life span of a fruit fly is only thirty days.

The reader may ask if flies have lungs, arteries and a heart. Yes, flies have hearts, in fact they have nine. In some way they are similar to your own heart for their purpose - a muscular pump that moves blood around the body, but in most ways the circulatory system of this insect is a little bizarre.

The principal heart is a muscular tube running down the middle of the fly under the skin. It is closed behind and extends forward through the breast to open behind the head. It has six slits in the abdominal portion, and beats at about 370 times per minute. The blood simply percolates back through the body until it reaches the belly to enter the slits again after several minutes. The blood of the fly carries no oxygen, as red blood cells do in your blood. Flies get their oxygen through a system of tubes connected directly to the atmosphere through 22 small holes along the sides of the fly's body. When you play hard, your heart must pump faster to supply more oxygen to your muscles, but the heart of a fly does not because oxygen flows directly through the other set of tubes.

While the principal heart helps move blood forward, most movement of blood in insects occurs by simply sloshing around in the open system, and sometimes the principle heart beats backwards, moving blood from the front to the back.

If experiments on mice and rabbits can tell us how we humans get cardiovascular disease, why not use fruit flies? I am of course joking. I admit that we may be able to get a quick answer, but it is unlikely that the answer is applicable for human beings, neither are the results from experiments on vegetarian rodents.

Sources

1. Lindsay S, Chaikoff IL. In Sandler M, Bourne GH (ed). Atherosclerosis and its origin. Academic Press, NY 1963, p 349-437.
Detweiler DK and others. Ann NY Acad Sci 1968;149:868-81.
Detweiler DK and others. Ann Gilbert C. Cornell Center for Mate-rials Research , Jan 18, 2006
If you want to read Carl S. Thummel's many papers about the fruit fly, go to www.ncbi.nlm.nih.gov/pubmed and write Thummel CS in the search field.

CHAPTER 2

The Diet Argument

Let me take you down,
'cause I'm going to Strawberry Fields
Nothing is real and nothing to get hung about
Strawberry Fields forever

Lennon/McCarthy

Saturated fat is the type of fat that dominates in animal food such as eggs, cream, meat and cheese and it is also abundant in palm oil and coconut oil. Today, too much saturated fat is considered just as dangerous to our arteries as are the greasy food leftovers destined for the sewer of our kitchen sink, but where is the evidence?

For several years skeptical scientists, including myself, have asked the experts on the Swedish National Food Administration about the scientific studies that encourage them to warn against saturated fat. Their usual answer has been that there are thousands of such studies, or they refer to the WHO guidelines,[1] said to have been written by the world's greatest experts.

The main argument in that document is that saturated fat raises cholesterol, but high cholesterol is not a disease. What we really want to know is, if we are shortening our life, or whether we are running a greater risk of suffering with a heart attack or a stroke, by eating too much saturated fat. To claim that it raises cholesterol is not enough; this is what scientists call a surrogate outcome. The proposition that high cholesterol is a risk factor for having a heart attack is only a hypothesis and, as I shall tell you later in this book, all the evidence shows that it is plainly wrong. In fact, high cholesterol is advantageous. For instance, more than twenty studies have shown that elderly people with high cholesterol live longer than elderly people with low cholesterol. The reader may be inclined to disbelieve me and I can certainly understand why, especially after everything we have been told about dangerous cholesterol, but it is true as you will learn soon.

Recently, the Swedish Food Administration published a list of seventy-two studies, which they claimed were in support of their warnings. Together with eleven colleagues I scrutinized the list and what we found was the following.

Eleven studies did not concern saturated fat at all.

Sixteen studies were indeed about saturated fat, but they were not in support.

Three reviews had ignored all contradictory studies.

Eleven studies gave partially or doubtful support.

Eight studies were reviews of experiments, where the treatment included not only a 'healthy' diet, but was combined with weight reduction, smoking cessation and physical exercise. So how did they know whether the small effect was due to less saturated fat or to something else? Furthermore, all of them had excluded several trials with a negative outcome.

Twenty-one studies were about surrogate outcomes. In most of the studies the authors claimed that saturated fat raises cholesterol. We should note that high cholesterol is not a disease.

Twelve studies were listed because they had shown that people on a diet, which included a high proportion of saturated fat and little carbohydrates, reacted more slowly to insulin than normally. From that observation, the authors claimed that saturated fat causes diabetes, but decreased insulin sensitivity is a normal reaction. When you cut the intake of carbohydrates radically, your metabolism is changed to spare blood glucose and it works by reducing your insulin sensitivity. That saturated fat produces diabetes is also contradicted by several experiments on patients with early or manifest type 2 diabetes. They have shown, that a diet with much saturated fat and little carbohydrates normalises the level of blood sugar and insulin and many of the patients are able to stop their medication.[2]

Another contradiction is, that for many years the consumption of saturated fat has decreased in many countries, while during the same time period we have seen a steady increase in the incidence of type 2 diabetes.

To their honour, the Food Administration also published another list that included eight studies which they said had contradicted their warnings. However, that list was incomplete, to put it mildly.

Why didn't they for instance include the many studies of the Masai people who have the lowest cholesterol ever measured in healthy people, although more than sixty percent of the calories in their food are derived from saturated fat?[3]

Why didn't they mention that cholesterol in people who gorge on saturated fat on average is on average no higher than in those who avoid it as if it was poison?

Why didn't they mention the thirty or more studies, which showed that patients who had suffered a myocardial infarction or a stroke had NOT eaten more saturated fat than healthy individuals.[4]

Why didn't they mention the nine studies which showed that patients who had suffered a stroke have eaten less saturated fat than healthy individuals?[5]

Why didn't they mention any of the numerous unsuccessful dietary trials? If a high intake of saturated fat causes heart disease, a reduction of the intake should be seen to reduce the risk. Until 1997 only nine such trials had been published and when all the results were collated in a so-called meta-analysis, a reduction of saturated fat was seen to have no effect. In a few of the trials fewer people died from myocardial infarction, but in just as many trials the mortality figures had increased.[4,6] Why is saturated fat still seen as a menace to our health today? Where is the evidence for this idea? The truth is that there is none. The truth is that the warnings against saturated fat are based upon data which has been manipulated.

Ancel Keys

Ask any scientist in this area to list the names of those who have created the cholesterol-diet-heart idea and nine out of ten would probably put the name of Ancel Keys on the top.

Keys had no clinical experience; he was an American professor in physiology. One of his first contributions in this area of science was a paper from 1953, where he stated that myocardial infarction was caused by too much fat in the diet. As an argument he used a diagram showing the association between the fat consumption and the mortality from heart disease in six countries. It looked very convincing, because all the observations were in accord. On top were the figures from the US; at the bottom were those from Japan. In America people ate five times more fat than in Japan, and heart mortality was fifteen times higher. The data from the other countries lay between those two data points, forming a beautiful curve starting in the lower left corner and ending in the upper right corner.[7]

What Keys was apparently unaware of was that the fat consumption figures, which he had collected from the FAO archives, did not reflect what people had actually eaten but it was a measure of the fat which had been available for consumption. This is an important point to make because much fat never reaches the human stomach. Some is eaten by rats, some is given to pet animals, and some is thrown away because of bad storage. In rich countries, where fat is considered synonymous with poison, most of the fat disappears in the kitchen or is cut away on the plate. In the poorer countries, where malnutrition and famine is a far greater problem than heart disease, all the fat is eaten.

The figures for the number of people who die from myocardial infarction is just as uncertain. These figures are provided by the World Health Organisation (WHO) archives and they are based upon death certificates.

Consider this: there is only room for one diagnosis on a death certificate. How often do you think that the diagnosis is correct on that piece of paper? In most countries, less than ten percent of dead people are examined by a coroner. Therefore the diagnosis reflects what the doctor believes is the cause of death. In a Swedish study Drs. George D Lundberg and Gerhard Voigt demonstrated that the diagnosis may often be wrong. They found that almost half of those whose cause of death was listed as a myocardial infarction according to the death certificate, had died from something else.[8]

The most serious error in Keys' paper was that he had excluded the data that didn't fit neatly into his hypothesis. I shall tell you more about that incident in the following paragraphs. Unfortunately, his paper is still used by the experts today to support the argument for their dietary guidelines, as is another one, called Seven Countries; published in 1972.[9] In that study, Keys had observed sixteen population groups in seven different countries and from his observations he concluded that one of the most important factors behind myocardial infarction was too much saturated fat in the diet.

The explanation, he said, is that if you eat too much saturated fat, your cholesterol goes up. This was what he and other researchers had seen in dietary experiments on healthy people. His message was swallowed by the rest of the world. Anyone who tries to question this sacred dogma today is considered to be a quack, although many studies have shown that it isn't true. Keys' idea was proved false by Raymond Reiser, an American professor in biochemistry, who pointed to several errors in these experiments.[10]

Instead of giving the test individuals natural saturated fat from animal food, many authors had used vegetable oils saturated by hydrogenation, a process that also produces trans fat, and today we know that trans fat does indeed cause cholesterol levels to rise. Additionally, when the cholesterol had increased, they had attributed the effect to high intakes of saturated fat, when it could just as easily have been due to low intakes of polyunsaturated fat.

Other researchers have studied this problem in recent times, but most of them have made similar errors. It is simply impossible to draw any valid conclusions about the effect of saturated fat alone from such trials.

What definitely puts the argument to rest is the outcome of modern dietary trials where scientists have used a diet low in carbohydrates with a high content of saturated fat to combat diabetes and/or obesity.[11] By avoiding bread, potatoes, cakes, cookies, candies and soft drinks these scientists have achieved amazing results. Even if the diet contained 20-50 percent of calories from saturated fat, there was no effect on the patients' blood cholesterol.[12]

Let us return to the Seven Countries paper. Apparently, very few have read the full 260 page report, because if you were to do that meticulously, as I have done, you will soon discover findings that are at odds with Keys' idea. For example, although the intake of saturated fat was almost equal in the two population groups from Turku and North Karelia in Finland, heart mortality was three times higher in North Karelia than in Turku. The saturated fat intake was also equal on two Greek islands, Crete and Corfu, but heart mortality was almost seventeen times higher on Corfu than on Crete.

Keys' lengthy report is loaded with irrelevant figures and tables and the many contradictory observations are easily overlooked. One of the findings was that while the intake of saturated fat was associated with heart mortality, it was not associated with the electrocardiographic findings. The people whose reading was pathological, had not eaten any more saturated fat than the others.

Who are we to believe? The local doctors who had written the death certificates, or the American experts who had evaluated all the ECGs?

More contradictions
During the eighties, American researcher Ronald Krauss found that the most useful risk marker, the best predictor of myocardial infarction among the blood lipids, wasn't the total amount of cholesterol in the

blood, neither was it the 'bad guy', LDL cholesterol. It was a special type of LDL particles, the small and dense ones. The most surprising finding was that if somebody ate a large amount of saturated fat, then the number of these small, dense LDL particles decreased.[13]

Isn't this just the opposite to what we would expect? Why should we avoid saturated fat if it lowers the risk of dying from a heart attack?

Good question, and this was also my question to Ronald Krauss when I met him in Chicago a few years ago. Krauss is not only a brilliant researcher; he is also a member of the committee, which writes the dietary guidelines for the American people.

Oh, you see, he answered, *the members of the committee do not always agree, and when we don't agree, we decide what to recommend by voting.*

I wonder if the committee voted when they discussed the study by the Indian researcher, Malhotra. For six years he had registered how many people had died from a heart attack among more than one million employees of the Indian railways. According to Malhotra's report; employees who lived in Madras had the highest mortality. It was six to seven times higher than in Punjab, the district with the lowest mortality, and the people from Madras also died at a much younger age. People in Punjab consumed almost seventeen times more fat than people from Madras and most of it was animal fat. In addition they also smoked much more than in Madras.[14]

I assume that many of the experts in the committee must have been skeptical of Malhotra's result: *How is that possible? How many of you believe in such nonsense? Raise your hands!*

Are dairy products dangerous?
Saturated fat is the dominating fat in milk, cream and cheese. This is why everybody praises the low fat dairy products, both for children and adults, but what does the science tell us?

In a British report, the authors had put together data from ten large studies including more than 400,000 men and women who had been studied for several years. What they found was that the number of heart attacks and strokes were smaller among those who had consumed the most dairy products, and a more recent Swedish study came up with the same result.[15]

A more reliable method
A relevant argument against such studies is this: what each participant says about their diet is not necessarily true.

Who will remember what food they ate yesterday and how much? Can we be confident that they would be eating similar food and similar amounts of that food next week or next year?

A better method is to analyse the amount of fatty acids which are present in the fat cells of the participants, because the number of the short saturated fatty acids reflects the intake of saturated fat during the previous weeks or months.[16] In at least nine studies researchers have used this method. In six of them the content was similar in patients with cardiovascular disease and in healthy individuals. In the rest, the patients had fewer short chain fatty acids, meaning that they had eaten less saturated fat.[17]

The answer from the Swedish Food Administration

I assume that you are curious to know how the Swedish Food Administration responded to our criticism. They did respond, but we couldn't find an answer to our questions about saturated fat. Indeed, we could not even find the term saturated fat in their text. Instead you could read statements such as *Our dietary guidelines are based on science... they are a synthesis of thousands of studies... they are based on the WHO guidelines.*

Can we rely on the WHO experts?

After almost twenty years of meticulous reading of the scientific reports, which are relevant to this issue, I haven't found any valid argument against saturated fat,[18] and I am not alone.[19] Instead, as you already know, I have found a large number of contradictory observations. Let's examine the WHO/FAO Expert Consultation[1] to see what the world's best experts have to say about it.

According to that paper *...the relationship between dietary fats and CVD (cardiovascular disease), especially coronary heart disease, has been extensively investigated, with strong and consistent associations emerging from a wide body of evidence.* This statement is followed by a reference to a consensus report from the Nutrition Committee of the American Heart Association.[20] The only evidence presented in that particular report are studies claiming that saturated fat raises cholesterol, and a single study claiming that intake of saturated fat may cause myocardial infarction.[21]

The first argument is not true, as you already know, and the second one is not true either. However, in the summary of that paper you can read the following: *our findings suggest that replacing saturated and trans unsaturated fats with unhydrogenated monounsaturated and polyunsaturated fats is more effective in preventing coronary heart disease in women than reducing overall fat intake.*

You would probably think that the study was a dietary trial, but it was not. It was a study of 80,000 healthy nurses and they had been studied for almost twenty years. At the start of the study and every year, the researchers from Harvard asked them about their usual diet. After fourteen years the diet of those who had suffered a heart attack was compared with the diet of those who had remained healthy. Thus, the term 'replacing' did not mean that they had replaced anything; it was the result of some complicated statistical calculations based upon the dietary information. The truth is this: on average, there were just as many heart attacks among those who had eaten the lowest intake of saturated fat and those with the highest intake; this fact appears clearly from the tables in their report. The same result also appeared within many other similar reports from the Harvard researchers.

A dietary U-turn?

Recently a new WHO-report was published. In cooperation with FAO, 28 experts had been selected to scrutinize the scientific literature about dietary fat.[22] This time the authors had looked at every type of study and realized that something was wrong. For example, in the section about saturated fat, two of the authors declare that *the available evidence from cohort and randomised controlled trials is unsatisfactory and unreliable to make judgements about and substantiate the effects of dietary fat on the risk of developing CHD.*

A most sensational statement indeed; at least for those who have listened to the warnings from the American Heart Association and the National Heart, Lung and Blood Institute. Nevertheless, don't be too happy, because the experts haven't changed their recommendations. In chapter 9 I shall tell you how they succeeded in turning white to black again.

Sources

1. Diet, nutrition and the prevention of chronic diseases. Report of a joint WHO/FAO expert consultation. WHO Technical Report Series 916, Geneva 2003.
2. Hays JH and others. Endocr Pract 2002;8:177-83.
   Arora SK, McFarlane SI. Nutr Metab 2005, 2:16-24.
3. Mann GV and others. J Atheroscler Res 1964;4:289-312.
4. Ravnskov U. J Clin Epidemiol 1998;51:443-460.
   Leosdottir M and others. J Cardiovasc Prev Rehabil 2007;14:701-6.
5. Takeya Y and others. Stroke 1984;15:15-23.
   McGee D and others. Int J Epidemiol 1985;14:97-105.

Omura T and others. Soc Sci Med 1987;24:401-7.

Gillman MW and others. JAMA 1997;278:2145-50.

Seino F and others. J Nutr Sci Vitaminol 1997;43:83-99.

Iso H and others. Circulation 2001;103:856-63.

Iso H and others. Am J Epidemiol 2003;157:32-9.

6. Hooper L and others. BMJ 2001;322:757-63.

Ravnskov U. BMJ 2002;324: 238.

7. Keys A.J Mount Sinai Hosp 1953;20:118-39.

8. Lundberg CD, Voigt GE. JAMA 1979;242;2328-30.

9. Keys A. Circulation 1970;41(suppl 1):1-211.

10. Reiser R. Am J Clin Nutr 1973;26:524-55.

11. Arora SK, McFarlane SI. Nutr Metab 2005;2:16-24.

Feinman RD, Volek JS. Scand Cardiovasc J 2008;42:256-63.

12. Brehm BJ and others J Clin Endocrinol Metab 2003;88:1617-23.

Foster GD and others. N Engl J Med 2003;348:2082-90.

Meckling KA and others. J Clin Endocrinol Metab 2004;89:2717-23.

Sharman MJ and others. J Nutr 2004;134:880-5.

Boden G and others.. Ann Intern Med 2005;142:403-11.

McAuley KA and others, Diabetologia 2005;48:8-16.

Yancy WS Jr and others. Nutr Metab 2005;2:34.

Noakes M and others. Nutr Metab 2006;3:7.

Volek JS and others. Lipids 2009;44:297-309.

13. Krauss RM and others. Am J Clin Nutr 2006;83:1025-31.

Dreon DM and others. Am J Clin Nutr 1998;67:828-36.

14. Malhotra SL. Br Heart J 1967;29:895-905.

15. Elwood PC and others. Eur J Clin Nutr 2004;58:718-24.

Holmberg S and others. Int J Environ Public Health 2009;6:2626-38.

16. Thomson M and others. Hum Nutr Appl Nutr 1985;39:443-55.

Smedman AE and others. Am J Clin Nutr 1999;69:22-9.

Wolk A and others. J Nutr 2001;131:828-33.

Rosell M and others. Int J Obes Relat Metab Disord 2004;28:1427-34.

Brevik A and others. Eur J Clin Nutr 2005;59:1417-22.

17. Scott RF and others. Am J Clin Nutr 1962;10:250-6.

Lang PD and others. Res Exp Med 1982;180:161-8.

Seidelin KN and others. Am J Clin Nutr 1992;55:1117-9.

Kirkeby K and others. Acta Med Scand 1972;192:513-9.

Wood DA and others. Lancet 1984;2:117-21.

Yli-Jama P and others. J Intern Med 2002;251:19-28.

Kark JD and others. Am J Clin Nutr 2003;77:796-802.

Clifton PM and others. J Nutr 2004;134:874-9.

Pedersen JI and others. Eur J Clin Nutr 2000;54:618-25.

18. Ravnskov U. J Clin Epidemiol 1998;51:443-60.

19. Olson R. J Am Diet Assoc 2000;100:28-32.

Taubes G. Science 2001;291:2535-41.

Weinberg SL. J Amer Coll Cardiol 2004;43:731-3.

German JB, Dillard CJ. Am J Clin Nutr 2004;80:550-9.

Okuyama H (ed). Prevention of coronary heart disease. From the cholesterol hypothesis to 6/3 balance. World Review of Nutrition and Dietetics, vol 96, Karger 2007

Mente A. Arch Intern Med 2009;169:659-69.

Ravnskov U. World Rev Nutr Diet 2009;100:90-109.

Siri-Tarion PW and others. Am J Clin Nutr 2010, doi:10.3945/ajcn.2009.27725

20. Kris-Etherton P and others. Circulation 2001;103:1034-9.
21. Hu FB and others. N Engl J Med 1997;337:1491-9.
22. Burlingame B and others (editors). Ann Nutr Metabol 2009;55:1-308.

CHAPTER 3
The Nobel Prize Argument

They had the best selection,
They were poisoned with protection
There was nothing that they needed,
Nothing left to find
They were lost in rock formations
Or became park bench mutations
On the sidewalks and in the stations
They were waiting, waiting

Neil Young

Less than one half percent of humans are born with much higher cholesterol than the rest of us. This abnormality, named familial hypercholesterolemia, is a genetic aberration. Those who inherit the abnormal gene from one of the parents is said to have heterozygous familial hypercholesterolemia. If both parents have familial hypercholesterolemia, half of their children may inherit the gene with the heterozygotic variant and there is a 25% risk that they will end up with familial hypercholesterolemia in a serious form, so-called homozygous familial hypercholesterolemia. The latter is extremely rare because the chance that two people with familial hypercholesterolemia will marry each other is of course very small.

All cells are able to take up cholesterol from the blood if their own production is insufficient. To do that they use the so-called LDL-receptor. However, in people with familial hypercholesterolemia, the receptor is malfunctioning and this is why their blood cholesterol is higher than in other people. This was what the world-famous American researchers Joseph Goldstein and Michael Brown discovered almost thirty years ago.

You can liken the receptor to an opening door in the cell wall. It is normally easy to open, but in people with familial hypercholesterolemia the hinge is a little crooked and because of this defect, it is more difficult to unlock so that less cholesterol can be taken into the cell.

In people with the homozygous variant no cholesterol is able to enter at all because our carpenter has forgotten to provide the door with a hinge.

For many years familial hypercholesterolemia has been considered as a serious disease, because people who die from a heart attack before age fifty usually have familial hypercholesterolemia. Because cholesterol is often present in large amounts within atherosclerotic lesions, Goldstein and Brown concluded that high cholesterol was the cause of atherosclerosis and myocardial infarction, not only in people with familial hypercholesterolemia but in all of us. Their discovery of the cholesterol receptor and their conclusion seemed to be so convincing that they were awarded the Nobel Prize in 1985.

Were they right? There is much evidence that they were not. Who would dare to question Nobel Prize laureates? Nevertheless – let me try.

First, the idea that most people with familial hypercholesterolemia die early from a heart attack is wrong. Previously, knowledge about familial hypercholesterolemia came from doctors, who saw the rare patient dying in his or her thirties or forties from a heart attack. A sad situation that became even worse when it appeared that some of their close relatives had died early as well. Therefore, the general opinion was that the risk of early heart disease was the same in all people with familial hypercholesterolemia.

When researchers started measuring cholesterol systematically in the general population, they found many healthy people with familial hypercholesterolemia living happily up to old age. From the data gathered in large Dutch and British studies including several thousands of such individuals, it appeared that, on average, they live just as long as others. More die from heart disease; but fewer die from cancer and other diseases. These calculations were based on a selection of those who had close relatives with premature heart disease, and the authors therefore assumed that the prognosis is even better for unselected individuals.[1]

An interesting study by a group of Dutch researchers showed that high cholesterol may even be advantageous. They found that before the year 1900 people with familial hypercholesterolemia lived longer than the average Dutchman, and because the most common cause of death then was an infectious disease, they drew the conclusion that high cholesterol protects against virus and bacteria.[2]

There is much support for that interpretation, because at least a dozen highly qualified research groups have shown that the lipoproteins, the molecules that we use for the transportation of cholesterol in our blood, have other important functions.

One of them is to bind and neutralize bacteria, viruses and their toxic products. Accordingly, low cholesterol is a risk factor for all kinds of infectious diseases.[3]

People with low cholesterol also have an increased risk of dying from diseases of the stomach, the guts and the lungs.[4] Most of these diseases are caused by bacteria or viruses. A relevant question is whether it is the infection that lowers cholesterol or the low cholesterol that predisposes to infectious diseases. You have probably guessed what the cholesterol experts suggest, but let us take a look at the facts.

To answer the question, more than 100,000 healthy individuals, living in the San Francisco area, were studied for fifteen years. It appeared that those, who had low cholesterol at the start had been admitted more often to hospital because of an infectious disease during the fifteen years.[5] This finding can't be explained away with the argument, that the infection had caused their cholesterol to go down. Evidently, low cholesterol, recorded at a time when these people were healthy, could not be caused by a disease with which they had not yet met.

The high cholesterol is innocent

One of the most interesting findings in familial hypercholesterolemia is that it is not their cholesterol level that determines who shall die early from heart disease. When researchers studied large numbers of people with familial hypercholesterolemia for several years, it appeared that those whose cholesterol was just a little higher than normal ran the same risk of heart disease as those whose cholesterol was twice as high or higher.[6]

The only conclusion, which can be drawn from these observations, is that high cholesterol is not a risk factor for myocardial infarction in cases of familial hypercholesterolemia. This is of course so very different from what we have learned about cholesterol in school, that even those who discovered it haven't understood it themselves.

There is another startling observation. If high cholesterol were the cause of atherosclerosis in these people, all of their arteries should be in danger, not only those going to the heart, because it is the same cholesterol rich blood that flows in all arteries, but this is not so. Even in those with the rare homozygous variant, the cerebral arteries are not more atherosclerotic than in normal people, although their cholesterol may be almost three times higher.[7]

Then what is the cause of cardiovascular disease in familial hypercholesterolemia? This is a relevant question, and there is a likely answer. Some of these people have inherited other genetic abnormalities.

They may, for example, have abnormally high levels of fibrinogen, factor VIII or prothrombin, molecules that are necessary actors in the coagulation process. If too little of these substances is present in the blood, bleedings may occur more easily; if there is too much then the blood clots more easily. The high concentration of each of these three is a risk factor for myocardial infarction in familial hypercholesterolemia, whereas high cholesterol is not.[8] This may also explain why atherosclerosis in familial hypercholesterolemia is located mainly to the arteries that are exposed to mechanical forces, such as the arteries of the heart and the legs, while premature atherosclerosis is absent in the arteries of the brain.

In spite of these contradictory findings, high cholesterol is still considered as the bad guy because since the introduction of the cholesterol reducing statins, young people with familial hyper-cholesterolemia die less often from heart disease. This is correct, but it cannot be the result of a reduction in cholesterol. Study after study has shown that the small effect achieved with these drugs is independent of the degree of cholesterol reduction. Those whose cholesterol is lowered only a little, gain the same benefit from such treatment as those whose cholesterol is lowered by more than fifty percent.

The explanation is probably that the statins have other, more useful qualities than reducing cholesterol. For example, statins have anticlogging effects on the blood, which evidently is useful for people who are born with too much fibrinogen, factor VIII or prothrombin in their blood. The result from a trial named ENHANCE even suggests that the cholesterol reducing effect is harmful. In that trial two cholesterol-reducing drugs were tested. Half of the participant group with familial hypercholesterolemia were given simvastatin, the other half were given simvastatin plus ezetimib (Vytorin®). The latter is a drug the only effect of which is to lower cholesterol.

Although cholesterol was reduced much more in the simvastatin/Vytorin group, the result was worse than in those who were treated with simvastatin alone. Obviously, cholesterol lowering is disadvantageous; the statins would probably have a better effect if they didn't lower cholesterol.[9]

Sources

1. Neil HA and others. Atherosclerosis 2005;179:293-7.
2. Sijbrands EJ and others. BMJ 2001;322:1019-23.
3. Ravnskov U. QJM 2003;96:927-34.
4. Jacobs D and others. Circulation 1992; 86:1046–60.

5. Iribarren C and others. Int J Epidemiol 1997; 26:1191–202.
6. Miettinen TA, Gylling H. Arteriosclerosis 1988;8:163-7.
    Hill JS and others. Arterioscler Thromb 1991;11:290-7.
    Ferrieres J and others.Circulation 1995; 92:290-5.
    Kroon AA and others. J Intern Med 1995;238:451-9.
    Hopkins PN and others. Am J Cardiol 2001;87:47-553.
    Jansen AC and others. Arterioscler Thromb Vasc Biol 2005;25:1475-81.
7. Postiglione A and others. Atherosclerosis 1991;90:23-30.
    Rodriguez G and others. Stroke 1994;25:831-6.
8. Jansen AC and others. Arterioscler Thromb Vasc Biol 2005;25:1475-81.
    Sugrue DD and others. Br Heart J 1985;53:265-8.
9. Kastelein JJP and others. N Engl J Med 2008;358:1431-43.

CHAPTER 4
The Risk Factor Argument

Some say it was radiation,
some say there was acid on the microphone,
Some say a combination
that turned their hearts to stone

Bob Dylan

In the introduction, I mentioned that just because something is associated with a disease it is not necessarily the cause; yellow fingers do not cause lung cancer, but repeatedly we are told the opposite. High cholesterol is considered to be a disease, and if we do not reduce it immediately, then a heart attack is waiting around the corner.

Of course, you cannot exclude it either. If high cholesterol really were causing atherosclerosis and myocardial infarction, high cholesterol would be dangerous for all of us. This is also what the experts have told us for many years, but nothing could be further from the truth.

Let us start with the Framingham study, whose directors were the first to air this idea. Do you know what they found when they examined the participants and their records thirty years after the start? I guess not, because very little, if anything is mentioned about it anywhere. The fact is that those who had high cholesterol and were older than forty-seven years of age when the project started lived just as long or longer than those with low cholesterol.[1] So, if you reach age forty-seven, it doesn't matter whether your cholesterol is high or low! If high cholesterol produces atherosclerosis, why is it a risk factor at age thirty, when little if any cholesterol is found in the arteries, but not after age forty-seven, the period of life where atherosclerosis accelerates?

Very few people die from a heart attack before that age, and most of them are diabetics or they have familial hypercholesterolemia. Almost all heart attacks occur in people older than forty-seven. If cholesterol has importance only for the very few, who have a heart attack before forty-eight, why should the rest of us worry about high cholesterol?

There was yet another surprise. Those whose cholesterol had decreased during these thirty years ran a greater risk of death than those whose cholesterol had increased. To cite the report: *For each 1 mg/dl drop of cholesterol there was an 11 percent increase in coronary and total mortality.*

Please read that again. Isn't it just the opposite of what we have been told repeatedly? Haven't we been told that the most important thing to do to prolong life is to lower our cholesterol?

But here, Framingham researchers tell us that those whose cholesterol went down died earlier than those whose cholesterol went up. Consider also, that among the people whose cholesterol went down, many had been treated with cholesterol lowering drugs. The abnormal results from Framingham do not stand alone either. Study after study has shown that high cholesterol is not a risk factor at all.

First, high cholesterol is not a risk factor for women. This was shown for the first time by a study from the National Heart, Lung, and Blood Institute almost twenty years ago. More than 80,000 women were studied for several years in six different countries. To their surprise, the authors found that those with low cholesterol run the same risk as those with high cholesterol.[2]

Have you ever heard or read that women need not worry about their high cholesterol? No, of course not and I have not yet met a doctor who knew it either. Have you ever heard a doctor telling you that if you are female, you shouldn't bother about high cholesterol? You should, preferably, be concerned if it is too low, because as I have mentioned in the previous section, high cholesterol protects you against infectious diseases.

Canadian researchers studied almost 5000 healthy middle-aged men for twelve years and came up with the same result.[3] They explained away their surprising finding by assuming that more than twelve years were necessary to see the harmful effects of high cholesterol. Obviously they had not yet read about the Framingham 30-year follow-up study.

The highest rate of heart attacks has probably occurred in Eastern Finland. Here, the Finnish researchers studied almost 2000 men for 1-5 years. During that time almost one hundred of these men had a myocardial infarction, but on average, their cholesterol was not higher than the others.[4]

In addition, study after study has shown that cholesterol is unimportant for those who have already had a heart attack.[5] Now consider that the strongest indication for cholesterol-lowering is the presence of established coronary disease.

Why should we lower cholesterol in high-risk patients if high cholesterol is not a risk factor for these people?

At least fifteen studies have shown that high cholesterol is not a risk factor for diabetic patients either.[6] In spite of that it is mandatory for the practising doctors in Sweden and most probably in many other countries, to treat all diabetics with cholesterol-lowering drugs, whether their cholesterol is high or low. Neither is it a risk factor for patients with renal disease[7] or, as you now know from the previous chapter, for people with familial hypercholesterolemia.

There are more exceptions, such as the Maori people, Polynesians who have migrated to New Zealand several hundred years ago. Maoris often die from heart attacks, but they do so whether their cholesterol is high or low.[8] Russian people are also an exception, because their risk is higher if their cholesterol is low rather than if it is normal.[9]

As high cholesterol is said to produce atherosclerosis, it should obviously be a risk factor for other diseases caused by atherosclerosis as well. However, high cholesterol is not a risk factor for stroke[10] or for arterial disease in the legs either.[11]

The most striking aberration is that all studies have shown that high cholesterol is a weak risk factor for old people; in most studies it was not a risk factor at all.[12] In a large study of old people living in the Bronx in New York, low cholesterol, not high, was a risk factor.[13]

Recently a gigantic study showed that cholesterol of patients with an acute myocardial infarction was, on average, lower than normal. I shall come back to that study later on.

The fact that high cholesterol is not a risk factor for old people should have stopped the cholesterol campaign long ago because in Sweden more than ninety percent of those who die from a myocardial infarction or a stroke have passed age 65. At least twenty studies have shown that old people with high cholesterol live longer than old people with low cholesterol.[14] In Japan even younger people benefit from high cholesterol. In a study including more than 20,000 people age 40 or older, total mortality was higher among those whose cholesterol was lower than 180 (4.65 mmol/) and highest among those with cholesterol below 140 (3.63 mmol/l).[15]

Sources

1. Anderson KM and others. JAMA 1987;257: 2176-80.
2. Jacobs D and others. Circulation 1992;86:1046-60.
3. Dagenais GR and others. Can J Cardiol 1990;6:59-65.
4. Salonen JT and others. Circulation 1991;84:129-39.

5. Shanoff HM and others. Can Med Ass J 1970;103:927-31.
    Gertler MM and others. Am J Med Sci 1964;247:145-55
    Frank CW and others. Circulation 1973;47:509-17.
    Mulcahy R and others. Br Heart J 1975;37:158-65.
    Khaw KT, Barrett-Connor E. J Cardiopulm Rehab 1986;6:474-80.
    Chester M and others. Br Heart J 1995;73:216-22.
    Behar S and others. Eur Heart J 1997;18:52-9.
6. Fontbonne A and others. Diabetologia 1989;32:300-4.
    Uusditupa MI and others. Am J Clin Nutr 1990;51:768-73.
    Fitzgerald AP, Jarrett RJ. Diabet Med 1991;8:475-80.
    Ford ES og DeStefano F. Am J Epidemiol 1991;133:1220-30.
    Laakso M and others. Circulation 1993;88:1421-30.
    Janghorbani M and others. J Clin Epidemiol 1994;47:397-405.
    Collins VR and others. Diabet Med 1996;13:125-32.
    Muggeo M and others. Circulation 1997;96:1750-4.
    Niskanen L and others. Diabetes Care 1998;21:1861-9.
    Hanninen J and others. Diabetes Res Clin Pract 1999;43:121-6.
    Biderman A and others.. Diabetes Care 2000;23:602-5.
    Forrest KY oa. Atherosclerosis 2000;148:159-69.
    Östgren CJ and others. Diabetes Care 2002;25:1297-302.
    Roselli della Rovere G and others.Nutr Metab Cardiovasc Dis 2003;13:46-51.
    Chan WB and others. Diabetes Metab Res Rev 2005;21:183-8.
7. Zoccali C and others. Lancet 2001;358:2113-7.
    Bellomo G and others. J Nephrol 2003;16:245-51.
8. Beaglehole R and others. BMJ 1980;1:285-7.
9. Shestov DB and others. Circulation 1993;88:846-53.
10. Prospective Studies Collaboration. Lancet 1995;346:1647-53.
11. Siitonen O and others. Acta Med Scand 1986;220:205-12.
    Uusitupa MI and others. Am J Clin Nutr 1990;51:768-73.
    Senti M and others. Circulation 1992;85:30-6.
    Aronow WS, Ahn C. Am J Cardiol 1994;3:995-7.
    Bainton D and others. Br Heart J 1994;72:128-32.
    Mölgaard J and others. Nutr Metab Cardiovasc Dis 1996;6:114-23.
    Wilt TJ and others. Arch Intern Med 1996;156:1181-8.
    Mowat BF and others. Atherosclerosis 1997;131:161-6.
    Katsilambros NL and others. Diabet Med 1996;13:243-6.
12. Siegel D and others. Am J Epidemiol 1987;126:385–9.
    Nissinen A and others. Ann Med 1989; 21:239–40.
    Weijenberg MP and others. J Clin Epidemiol 1994; 47:197–205.
    Simons LA and others. Aust NZ J Med 1996; 26:66–74.
    Weijenberg MP and others. Am J Epidemiol 1996; 143:151–8.
    Räihä I and others. Arterioscl Thromb Vasc Biol 1997; 17:1224–32.
    Simons LA and others. Atherosclerosis 2001; 159:201–8.
    Abbott RD and others. Ann Epidemiol 2002; 12:173–81.
13. Krumholz HM and others. JAMA 1994;272:1335-40.
14. Kozarevic D and others. Am J Epidemiol. 1981;114:21-8.
    Rudman D and others. J Am Geriatr Soc 1987;35:496-502.

Siegel D and others. Am J Epidemiol 1987;126:385-99.

Forette B and others. Lancet 1989;1:868-70.

Staessen J and others. J Hypertens 1990;8:755-61.

Harris T and others. J Clin Epidemiol 1992;45:595-601.

Casiglia E and others. Eur J Epidemiol 1993;9:577-86.

Weverling-Rijnsburger AW and others. Lancet 1997; 350:1119–23.

Jonsson A and others. Lancet 1997;350:1778-9.

Räihä I and others. Arterioscler Thromb Vasc Biol 1997;17:1224-32.

Behar S and others. Eur Heart J 1997;18:52-9.

Fried LP and others. JAMA 1998;279:585-92.

Chyou PH, Eaker ED. Age Ageing 2000;29:69-74.

Schatz IJ and others. Lancet 2001;358:351-5.

Weverling-Rijnsburger AW and others. Arch Intern Med 2003;163:1549-54.

Onder G and others. Am J Med 2003;115:265-71.

Casiglia E and others. J Intern Med 2003;254:353-62.

Psaty BM and others. J Am Geriatr Soc 2004;52:1639-47.

Ulmer H and others. J Womens Health 2004;13:41-53.

Schupf N. J Am Geriatr Soc 2005;53:219-26.

Akerblom JL and others. Age Ageing 2008;37:207-13.

15. Kirihara Y and others. J Lipid Nutr 2008;17:67-78

Ogushi Y and others. World Rev Nutr Diet 2009;100:63-70.

CHAPTER 5
An Argument to Forget

There's a code of silence, that we don't dare speak
There's a wall between and the river's deep
We keep pretending that there's nothing wrong
But there's a code of silence, and it can't go on

Bruce Springsteen

If cholesterol circulating in the blood tends to settle in the arterial wall and produce atherosclerosis only because the blood contains more of it than normally, then people with high cholesterol should, on average, be more atherosclerotic than people with low cholesterol. This is pure logic and this is also what we have been told again and again. In 1953, Ancel Keys wrote the following: *It is a fact that a major characteristic of the sclerotic artery is the presence of abnormal amounts of cholesterol in that artery, and he added: This cholesterol is derived from the blood.*[1] No proofs and no arguments were offered by Keys, nor by his many followers. The cholesterol comes from the blood, and what is meant by that is that it goes into the arterial wall because there is too much of it in the blood. Even today, high cholesterol is seen as the starting point for the inflammatory processes within the arterial wall, the result of which is the atherosclerotic plaque.

But where is the evidence? Where are the scientific studies that clearly and definitely have shown that it is true? The answer is simple; there are none. On the contrary, study after study has shown that this idea cannot be true. Let us take a short look at some of them.

The Japanese dilemma
On average, people in the US have much higher cholesterol than have the Japanese people. It follows that Americans must be more atherosclerotic than Japanese people. Fifty years ago researchers from both countries became curious and decided to see if it was true. They examined the aorta, the main artery of the body, in about one thousand dead American and Japanese people.

To their surprise they found that the Japanese people's arteries were as atherosclerotic as the Americans'.[2] In a similar study of more than 7000 American and Japanese people, the latter were even more atherosclerotic than Americans.[3]

To use mean values from a whole country, as in these examples, is of course liable to bias. A better way is to compare the degree of atherosclerosis with blood cholesterol in each individual, or to compare the amount of cholesterol in the artery wall with the concentration of cholesterol in the blood. This has indeed been done several times, and each time with the same result.

The first such study was performed in 1936 by the pathologist Kurt Landé and the biochemist Warren Sperry from New York.[4] They examined the arteries of people, who had died suddenly as victims of homicide, suicide or because of an accident. No association was seen. Those with low cholesterol were just as atherosclerotic as those with high cholesterol.

If those people, who were to promote the cholesterol hypothesis later on, had read that paper they would probably have dropped the idea at once. Landé's and Sperry's findings have been confirmed by colleagues from Canada, Guatemala, India and Australia.[5] After an examination of almost one thousand patients during surgery, American and world-renowned heart surgeon Michael DeBakey came up with the same message: *Atherosclerosis has nothing to do with the concentration of cholesterol in the blood.* [6]

Angiography

With the arrival of bypass surgery, coronary angiography has assumed great importance. On the x-ray pictures, shadows show how much the vessels have been narrowed. If we know the cholesterol values of patients studied in this way, we are able to see if people with rough and irregular arteries have higher cholesterol than people with smooth ones. A large number of radiologists from America have performed such studies, and all of them have emphasized the importance of cholesterol in the narrowing of arteries. However, their reports offer only statistical formulas that most readers are unable to interpret. People familiar with statistics can tell you that the associations found in these studies were extremely weak.

The idea that blood cholesterol determines whether atherosclerosis will appear or not is also in conflict with a number of longterm x-ray studies.

According to conventional wisdom, atherosclerosis increases if cholesterol goes up, and it decreases, or at least it should not increase, if cholesterol goes down.

Any type of association between an increase in the suspected causal factor, in this case cholesterol, and a worsening of the disease, in this case atherosclerosis, is called exposure-response. The presence of exposure-response in which the change in the suspected causal factor, here I mean blood cholesterol, and the change in the incidence of the disease both go in the same direction, and only in that direction, suggests that the factor in question is the cause of the disease.

However, it is not sufficient, by itself, to prove causality because an innocent risk marker may go in the same direction as the real cause and thus introduce a false impression of an exposure-response. There is exposure-response between yellow fingers and lung cancer for example; the more discolored the fingers are, the greater the risk, but it is of course not the yellow fingers that cause lung cancer. Absence of an exposure-response definitely disproves causality, however. If non-smokers got lung cancer more often than smokers, we could definitely conclude that smoking is not the cause of lung cancer. Similarly, if atherosclerosis become worse if cholesterol goes down then we can bin the cholesterol hypothesis. Studies of exposure-response are therefore of great importance.

Among the first people who studied the inside of the coronary vessels with that question in mind were Charles Bemis and his co-workers from Peter Bent Brigham Hospital in Boston.[7] When they performed a second angiography two years after the first one, those whose cholesterol went down had become more atherosclerotic, than those whose cholesterol went up. It should of course have been the opposite.

Similar results have been achieved by other researchers.[8] Some of them found no difference, but none of them found the opposite. In one of the papers the authors concluded that *medical treatment directed toward secondary prevention* (meaning cholesterol lowering in patients with heart disease) *may be unsuccessful in retarding or reversing the development of progressive arterial lesions and their clinical consequences.*

Electron beam tomography

Bemis, his many colleagues and their results appear to be unknown today. Perhaps many researchers are unwilling to use their precious time reading old papers. Probably they think that they are less reliable because their colleagues hadn't access to the many sophisticated methods we use today.

One of them is called electron beam tomography, a technique that depicts calcified atherosclerotic plaques whether they are located on the inner surface of the artery or they are buried inside its wall.

With this technique two American researchers examined the coronary arteries in hundreds of patients. Again, no association was found. The arteries of those with low LDL-cholesterol were, on average, just as calcified as the arteries of those with the highest levels.[9]

Sources

1. Keys A. J Mount Sinai Hosp 1953;20:118-39.
2. Gore I and others. Am J Clin Nutr 1959;7:50-4.
3. Resch JA and others. Geriatrics 1969;November:111-32.
4. Landé KE, Sperry WM. Arch Pathol 1936;22:301-12.
5. Paterson JC and others. Circulation 1963;27:229-36.
   Mathur KS and others. Circulation 1961;23:847-52.
   Marek Z and others. Am Heart J 1962;63:768-74.
   Schwartz CJ and others. Br Heart J 1965;27:731-9.
   Méndez J, Tejada C. Am J Clin Nutr 1967;20:1113-7.
   Rhoad GG and others. Lab Invest 1978;38:304-11.
6. Garrett HA and others. JAMA 1964;189:655-9.
7. Bemis CE m.fl. Circulation 1973;47:455-64.
8. Kramer JR and others. Am Heart J 1983;105:134-44.
   Kimbiris D and others. Am J Cardiol 1974;33:7-11.
   Shub C m.fl. Mayo Clin Proc 1981;56:155-60.
9. Hecht HS, Superko HR. JACC 2001;37:1506-11.

CHAPTER 6
The Trial Argument

Let me tell you how it will be
There's one for you, nineteen for me
'cause I'm the taxman, yeah, I'm the taxman

George Harrisson

Many of my colleagues consider me to be a crank. How can Ravnskov ignore or deny the importance of high cholesterol? Doesn't he know that experiments, which are carried out on human beings, are the best way to prove causality? Doesn't he know that cholesterol lowering drugs are able to prevent all types of cardiovascular disease?

Experiments are the best way to establish causality, this is true. If we were able to prevent atherosclerosis and its consequences by only reducing the amount of cholesterol in the blood, it would indeed be the strongest proof. The problem is that we can't. Here most doctors and researchers probably shake their head; Ravnskov is hopelessly ignorant.

I am not; let me explain.

How to perform an experiment on human beings
As atherosclerosis and myocardial infarction may hit us whether our diet is fat or lean, and whether our cholesterol is high or low, there must be something wrong with the cholesterol hypothesis. Up to this point I have only written about observations, and in science observations are less reliable than experiments. The crucial question is this; what will happen if we reduce people's cholesterol?

To learn what happens when we lower cholesterol we must include untreated people in our experiment. These people must, on average, have the same risk of myocardial infarction at the start as those we treat. This means, on average, that they have the same cholesterol, the same smoking habits, the same body weight and so forth. In very large studies, risk factors usually become evenly distributed by chance, provided that the study participants are assigned randomly to the two study groups.

Experiments where the participants are allocated randomly to two or more study groups are called controlled, randomized trials.

A further complication is that many trials have not been unifactorial, meaning that the only treatment has been to lower cholesterol. In several trials, the directors had instructed the participants to stop smoking, to take regular exercise, and to reduce their body weight as well. This is called a multifactorial trial, and if benefit is achieved, it is impossible to know which of the factors was responsible. Some of these trials have lowered the risk of heart disease, and surprise, surprise, these are the trials most often cited as support.

The importance of being blind

To be convincing, a clinical trial should be conducted blindly, meaning that the patients shouldn't know whether they belong to the treatment group or to the control group. In the best experiments, the so-called double-blind trials, not even the doctors know. Unfortunately most of the older trials were neither single or double blind, and some of them were even multifactorial.

In 1992 several authors had analysed the combined result of all of the trials in a so-called meta-analysis. As all of them were incomplete because the authors had excluded some of the unsuccessful trials, I decided to perform my own, which was published in British Medical Journal that year. As very few of the trials had been conducted in the correct way, I included all of them, whether they were uni or multifactorial and whether they were open or blinded, with the proviso that they were both controlled and randomized.[1]

The design of my review was obviously advantageous for the cholesterol campaign. Despite this, when all results were taken together, the number who had died from a heart attack was the same in the treatment and the control groups. Worse was that if all causes of death were taken together, more had died in the treatment groups. Although my analysis was published in one of the world's most respected medical journals, it made absolutely no impact on the medical community. In the cholesterol-reducing world, scientists only take notice of trials with a positive outcome, or more correctly, with an allegedly positive outcome. In my previous books, I have given many details about these trials. Let it suffice here to briefly mention a few of the most important ones.

The North Karelia project

Several of the most often cited trials have been performed in Finland. This country was also one of the first to introduce cholesterol reduction measures in the general population because Finland was a nation with the highest mortality from myocardial infarction. The mortality was especially high in the province called North Karelia and it increased year by year up to the 1960s. The health authorities were concerned. To them, it was self-evident that the cause was high cholesterol, because in Finland cholesterol levels were also higher than in most other countries, and the highest values were noted in North Karelia.

A team of doctors and scientists headed by Professor Pekka Puska at the University of Kuopio decided to do something about the problem. They chose to start in North Karelia. To see whether their efforts were of benefit, they used the population in Kuopio as a control group, because in Kuopio the mortality was just as high. In 1972, a public health campaign began throughout North Karelia. In the media, on posters, at public meetings and through campaigns in schools and work places people were told to stop smoking, to reduce their cholesterol and to avoid saturated fat. In Kuopio people were allowed to live as they had traditionally lived.

Five years later the number of heart attacks among North Karelian men had decreased a little each year.[2] The total mortality had also declined and the directors of the campaign were confident that the trend would continue. Apparently, cholesterol lowering was beneficial, and the promising result is also why the North Karelia Project is used as an example of a successful trial. In a following chapter I shall tell you why the conclusion of the experts was too hasty.

Helsinki Heart Study

Another frequently cited trial is the Helsinki Heart Study. The investigators advised more than 4000 healthy, middle-aged men with high cholesterol to quit smoking, to exercise and to lose weight. Half of them received the drug gemfibrozil (Lopid®, Jezil®, Gen-Fibro®), a cholesterol reducing medicine from a group of drugs named the fibrates and still used today; the others were given a placebo drug.

As in most other trials heart mortality was unchanged but there was a fall in the number of nonfatal heart attacks.[3] According to the hypothesis, cholesterol is dangerous because it generates atherosclerosis. If this were true, then the risk of other diseases caused by atherosclerosis should also have been reduced.

In the tables of the early trials, the reader will often see that the number of 'other cardiovascular diseases' has increased a little, and so it was here as well. If all cardiovascular diseases were put together, the difference between the two groups became much smaller and could just as well have been due to chance. In addition, the treatment produced some unpleasant side effects. During the first year many more in the treatment group were operated on for ailments of the gastrointestinal tract. The question is whether you would prefer to have an operation on your stomach or gall bladder, or sustain a nonfatal heart attack, because the sum of heart attacks and operations was almost identical in the two groups.

The Oslo trial

Another often-cited study came from Oslo, Norway. Here, Dr. Ingvar Hjermann and his team advised half of around 1200 middle-aged men, mostly smokers with high cholesterol, to avoid saturated fat and to stop smoking.[4] After five years it was clear that nineteen had died from a heart attack in the treatment group against thirty-five in the control group. Apparently a benefit, but did the experiment really prove that a faulty diet causes myocardial infarction? The authors had admitted that if dietary advice had been the only treatment, their result would not have been statistically significant but this is not the end of the story. I shall come back to this trial in the next chapter.

Greg Brown

Clinical experiments on thousands of individuals are labour-intensive and very expensive, but there is a shortcut. Instead of counting the number who die, we can evaluate the vascular changes on x-ray images which are taken some years apart. If the mean diameter of a coronary artery increases, or if it decreases less than in untreated patients, it is taken as a sign of improvement. Angiographic trials are much cheaper because fewer test individuals and shorter test periods are necessary.

Until 1990 a number of such trials had been published with questionable results. They were explained by the argument that cholesterol had not been lowered sufficiently well, but the statins changed the situation. One of the first angiographic statin trials was conducted by Greg Brown and his team from Washington, DC. It is also one of the most cited.[5]

In this particular trial cholesterol was reduced in men with heart disease and high cholesterol; in three ways.

One-third of the men were given colestipol (Lestid®) and nicotinic acid, another third were treated with colestipol and one of the new statin drugs lovastatin (Mevacor®) and the rest were given a placebo drug. Indeed, cholesterol went down; in the first group by thirty-three per cent, in the statin group by almost fifty percent.

The width of the coronary arteries was measured using x-ray images magnified by five times. Magnification was necessary because the average vessel diameter in the first group increased by a mere 0.04 mm only, in the second it decreased by 0.002 mm and in the control group by 0.05 mm. These small differences were statistically significant, and Brown and his colleagues therefore considered their trial as a success.

But a decrease of the diameter, seen in the second group, the group, where cholesterol was lowered the most, is not an improvement, even though the diameter in the control group had decreased even more. The authors offered no comment about that. In fact, the title of their paper said the opposite: *Regression* (meaning improvement) *of coronary artery disease as a result of intensive lipid-lowering therapy.*

The use of laboratory changes rather than the number of deaths as a measure of treatment effect is a surrogate outcome. It is not self-evident that changes seen on x-ray pictures can be translated into clinical effects. It is also questionable whether a widening of a coronary vessel observed on x-ray is the same as the regression of atherosclerosis.

Artery walls are equipped with smooth muscle cells. When they contract, the artery narrows, and when they relax, it widens. Contraction is induced by mental stress, anxiety, exposure to cold and even a sustained handgrip. The latter effect was studied six years earlier by Brown himself. He found that a handgrip sustained for a few minutes was followed by a 35 percent decrease in the vessel diameter.[6] Heart patients often take drugs that relax the coronary arteries, and a further problem is that when atherosclerosis starts, arteries do not become narrower, they widen. The atherosclerotic plaque must occupy more than thirty percent of the arterial wall before the artery starts narrowing.[7]

How could Brown know, which of these factors were responsible for the minimal changes seen? Was it an effect of the cholesterol reduction treatment? Was it the patients' usual medical treatment, which had been changed? Could the patients have been reasonably relaxed? Is it possible that they may have squeezed the nurse's hand more or less tightly? Were the changes due to the different stages of atherosclerosis growth?

Brown and his co-workers were aware of some of the problems. For example, they had tried to duplicate the medical treatment accurately.

However, they didn't mention anything about duplicating the patients' stress feelings or the degree of their squeezing the nurse's hand.

What I mention here is of course relevant for many other angiographic trials. It is simply impossible to derive meaningful results from such studies.

No exposure-response

Even if a widening of the artery reflects an improvement, it cannot have anything to do with cholesterol.

How do I know that?

From the results of the many angiographic trials, of course. If a decrease in cholesterol should explain the widening of the arteries, a more pronounced lowering of cholesterol should widen them more. In other words, we would expect to find an exposure-response. To see if this was the case in the angiographic trials, I searched for all trial reports where the authors had calculated exposure-response. I found a total of twenty-two, and with one exception all of them agreed: there was no exposure-response.[8] This is not a minor aberration; as I have stressed above, absence of exposure-response is simply the strongest proof that blood cholesterol has nothing to do with atherosclerosis.

Now let me tell you about the trial that became the official start of the cholesterol campaign and the National Cholesterol Education program.

LRC

This trial was initiated in the seventies by The National Heart, Lung, and Blood Institute and named the Lipid Research Clinics Coronary Primary Prevention Trial, or LRC.[9] Cholesterol was measured in almost one-third of a million middle-aged men, and only those with the highest cholesterol were included, a total of 4000. After a few weeks of dietary indoctrination, half of them were started on a new cholesterol-lowering drug cholestyramine (Questran") while the other half received a placebo.

After 7-8 years the difference in the numbers of heart attacks was so small that it could only be attributed to chance, and the difference in number of deaths from all causes was even smaller. Of half a million screened men, life was prolonged for only five. A few less died from a heart attack; a few more died from other causes.

Nevertheless, this trial was considered as the final proof that high cholesterol was harmful and should be reduced, because the benefit regarding nonfatal myocardial infarction was a little better.

Now, it was said that cholesterol should be reduced, not only in young and middle-age men with extremely high cholesterol, such as those who had been studied in the LRC trial, but also in women, children and old people. Obviously the committee had forgotten the many previous unsuccessful trials, and more would soon follow. Let me just mention a few of them.

The Coronary Drug Project

In the first mega-trial, The Coronary Drug Project, five different cholesterol lowering treatments were studied, but three of the treatment groups were stopped prematurely because it was evident that the treatment had increased mortality instead of decreasing it. Two groups completed the treatment, but at the end of the trial the number of fatal and non-fatal myocardial infarctions in the treatment group did not differ from the number in the control group. Besides, the drugs used, clofibrate (Atromidin®) and nicotinic acid, produced many unpleasant adverse effects.[10]

The WHO trial

Four years before the consensus conference the report from another large study, the WHO trial was published. Again clofibrate was tested. The number of non-fatal heart attacks had decreased, but the number of fatal ones had increased. In total 128 people died in the clofibrate group but only 87 in the placebo group.[11]

MRFIT

Two years later researchers from the National Heart, Lung, and Blood Institute published the final report from the Multiple Risk Factor Intervention Trial, or MRFIT. To find 12,000 middle-aged, healthy men especially prone to heart disease more than 360,000 had been recruited. Half of them were instructed to quit smoking, to exercise, to lower their blood pressure and to eat a 'healthy' diet. Every four months the subjects were called in for blood sampling and for counseling sessions to determine whether they had understood the guidelines. The trial continued for 7-8 years and the directors were satisfied with the risk factor changes. The difference in number of deaths between the two groups was trivial, however. Fewer in the treatment group had died from myocardial infarction, but more had died from other causes. In total, 265 had died in the treatment group, but only 260 in the untreated control group.[12]

The Miettinen trial

In Finland a trial was performed by Tatu Miettinen and his co-workers. It included about 1200 middle-aged male business executives who were considered to be overweight, with high cholesterol and high blood pressure. Half of them were given the same advices as in MRFIT. If their cholesterol or blood pressure were too high, they were also treated with various blood pressure and cholesterol-lowering drugs. Again the risk factors changed satisfactorily, but in spite of that twice as many died in the treatment group as in the control group.[13]

The statin trials

The many unsuccessful trials did not change anything, probably because more effective cholesterol-lowering drugs were introduced. The general opinion was that the trial failures were because the cholesterol hadn't been lowered sufficiently.

The new drugs, the statins, inhibit the body's production of many important substances, one of which is cholesterol, and they do it effectively. Today it is possible to cut cholesterol by half.

The outcome of the statin trials is seemingly a victory for the cholesterol hypothesis. However, when we take a closer look at the results, it is obvious that the cholesterol lowering effect is unimportant and actually a disadvantage. Furthermore, the benefits are trivial and apply only to certain small patient groups. In addition, the directors of the trials and the drug companies have succeeded in exaggerating the benefits and belittling the side effects. They do it using statistical manipulation and clever criteria for selection of the test individuals and by introducing new, generous limits to what are considered to be normal laboratory results. Today most doctors believe that statin treatment is a harmless way to eradicate mankind's worst enemy, the cardiovascular diseases. In the following paragraphs, I shall show that this is far from reality. Let me briefly describe the trials, which are most often used as arguments for cholesterol reduction.

Statin experiments on high-risk patients

One of the first was The Scandinavian Simvastatin Survival Study, or 4S. It was published in 1994, and it was the first cholesterol lowering trial that had succeeded in reducing both nonfatal and fatal myocardial infarction, as well as total mortality.[14] The steering committee and monitoring staff included employees from Merck, and all analyses and data from the trial were processed without outside supervision at their laboratories in the US. Altogether 4444 patients were treated, half of them with the drug simvastatin, half with a placebo pill.

Four to five years later 8.5 percent had died from a heart attack in the control group compared with 5 percent in the treatment group. The improvement included men only; the number of women who died from a heart attack was equal in both groups, or to be more accurate, a few more women died in the statin group although there were other benefits. The number of nonfatal heart attacks was lowered a little more and the number of strokes was also reduced.

Curiously, in the following, even larger HPS trial the results were only half as good as in 4S study, although it was the same drug, the same dose and the same type of participants, and cholesterol was reduced just as much. However, it is the figures from the 4S trial that are used for the marketing process. It is also the trial that the advocates of cholesterol lowering refer to when advocating statin treatment because the results of all the following trials were less favourable. In the LIPID trial for instance, the difference in heart mortality was a mere 1.9 percentage points,[16] and in other trials even less.[17] In most trials the total number of deaths was unchanged. Fewer died from myocardial infarction, while more died from other causes.

When I was practicing medicine and a patient with heart disease asked me to prescribe a statin drug, I could tell him about the benefit in the following way: As you are sixty years old, your chance to be alive in the next six years is about ninety percent. If you take a statin tablet every day you can increase your chance to ninety-two percent, but then you expose yourself to many unpleasant side effects.

Statin experiments on healthy people

Today high cholesterol is considered to be a disease, and as the American cholesterol experts lower the upper limit for what they consider to be normal every five years, most healthy people on this planet will soon become patients. Let us therefore have a closer look at some of the experiments where cholesterol has been lowered in healthy people with high cholesterol.

The first one, the EXCEL trial, is little known. It was conducted by a large number of American clinics and research institutions together with Merck, the drug manufacturer. More than 8,000 healthy individuals (named 'patients' in the trial reports) received one of four different doses of lovastatin (Mevacor®) or a placebo.[18]

There are two reasons why so few researchers refer to that trial; it was concluded after only one year, and the result was nothing to boast about. I shall return to that particular trial later.

The WOSCOPS trial was not much better. It had included more than 6,000 healthy middle-aged men and the drug on trial was pravastatin (Pravachol®). After five years 1.6% had died from myocardial infarction in the control group, and 1.2% among those treated with pravastatin.[19] This small difference, a mere 0.4 percentage points, wasn´t even statistically significant; it could as well have been due to chance.

In spite of that the WOSCOPS trial is used as an argument for lowering high cholesterol in healthy people. They do it by expressing the benefit in another way; they say that mortality was reduced by twenty-five percent. How can they do that? Because the difference of 0.4 percentage points is twenty-five percent of 1.6.

A similar experiment was the Air Force/Texan Coronary Atherosclerosis Prevention Study, or AFCAPS/TexCAPS. Head of the trial was the former president of the American Heart Association, Professor Antonio Gotto. Three of the co-authors were employees at Merck, the company whose drug lovastatin (Mevacor®) was tested in more than 6,000 healthy people with normal cholesterol.[20]

After five years 2.4% had died in the treatment group and 2.3% had died in the control group. The trial directors claimed that the primary target in this trial was not to lower mortality, but to reduce the number of all sorts of heart attacks. They also said that the number of heart attacks was lowered by 37%. This figure is the difference between 3.5%, the number in the treatment group, and 5.5%, the number in the control group, and the difference of 2 is 37% of 5.5.

Statin experiments on healthy people with low cholesterol

Is it possible to prevent heart attacks even in healthy people with low cholesterol? This seems a curious question because the bad guy is said to be high cholesterol. Why should we lower cholesterol in healthy people if their own cholesterol is already low?

The answer from the cholesterol prophets is that cholesterol lowering with statins is beneficial for all of us, whether it is high or low. Another reason, so they say, is that there is yet another risk factor of which to be afraid. It is a normal protein molecule in our blood named C-reactive protein, or CRP for short. The concentration of that protein is elevated in all kinds of inflammatory diseases, as well as in atherosclerosis, because atherosclerosis starts as an inflammation in the arterial wall.

What had been seen previously was that statin treatment lowered not only cholesterol but also CRP. The consequence of this idea is that most of us should start taking a statin drug from the age of two and for the rest of our life. It has even been suggested that statins should be put into the drinking water.

To test the idea, another new statin trial named JUPITER, was started.[21] It included almost 18,000 healthy men and women with elevated CRP. It can't have been too easy to find so many healthy people with high CRP because as mentioned, high CRP is mostly seen in patients with an inflammatory disease, and such patients were excluded from the trial. Thus, the trial included healthy people with a CRP, which was too high for reasons unknown. To find a sufficiently large number of such people it was necessary to conduct the trial at 1315 different sites in 26 countries. Half of the participants were given rosuvastatin (Crestor®) Astra-Zeneca's statin drug, and Astra-Zeneca had also paid for the trial.

The trial was stopped after less than two years because, as the directors declared, there were significantly more people who had died in the untreated group. For the first time a statin trial had succeeded in lowering mortality in healthy people, and by almost 20 percent. The directors were excited, as were the press. In the Wall Street Journal for instance a headline said: *Cholesterol Drug Cuts Heart Risk in Healthy Patients*, and similar optimistic verbiage was used in other newspapers. It was easy to understand that everybody could avoid heart disease. Obviously nobody had observed that the participants did not represent common people; they belonged to a rare variant of human beings, healthy people with high CRP.

Let us also have a look at the absolute lowering of mortality. In the control group 247 people had died, but only 198 in the treatment group. Thus, if you have passed the age of fifty and belong to this unusual variant of the human race, your chance of being alive in two years without treatment is 97.2 %. You can increase that chance to 97.8% if you take a Crestor tablet every day. Hooray!

However, at the same time you have an increased risk of getting diabetes, because among the untreated participants 216 got diabetes, whereas in the treatment group the number was 270. In other words, 49 fewer died but 54 more got diabetes.

You could also say that to save the life of one of these rare people every year you have to treat about 330 healthy people, none of whom would gain any benefit; on the contrary they run a considerable risk of developing unpleasant side-effects.

A statin experiment on old patients

It is often said that the statins are effective for people of all ages. It is true that a small cardiovascular benefit has been seen in old, high-risk patients, but there is a problem. Let us look at the PROSPER trial, a study that only included such people. As in the previous trials no effect was seen concerning mortality; fewer died from myocardial infarction, but more died from cancer and with statistically significance.[22] The directors were eager to explain away their unpleasant result. How they succeeded with that is the issue of another chapter.

The statins cure everything

Statins are said to be useful against more than heart disease, e.g. cancer, lung disease, heart failure, hip fractures and much more. The way in which researchers have studied these alleged benefits is confounded with a serious error. As an example I shall analyse the allegation that statin treatment prevents Alzheimer's disease. The idea goes against common sense. Today we know that not only is the brain the cholesterol-richest organ in the body; cholesterol is also vital for its function, because the creation of nerve impulses demands a steady production of cholesterol.

First, the evidence for this alleged effect does not come from trials. Instead, researchers have counted the number of patients with Alzheimer's disease among people with low cholesterol and among people treated with statins. Because the upper limit for normal cholesterol has been lowered increasingly, we can be confident that the untreated people's cholesterol was not only low, it was very low. The fact that most Alzheimer patients were identified in this low-cholesterol group is seen as a proof that statin treatment prevented those in the other group.

What has been forgotten is that low cholesterol is a frequent finding in people with various types of mental disturbances. For example, people whose cholesterol is lower than 200 are much more likely to decline in functional performance tests such as walking, turning around and dressing themselves.[23] In addition, people with high cholesterol develop Parkinson's disease and dementia less often than people with low cholesterol.[24,25] Detailed records of the ability of people to learn, to reason, to concentrate and to organize their thoughts have also shown that, on average, the smartest people have the highest cholesterol.[26] That statins should prevent Alzheimer's disease is also contradicted by the finding that people with high cholesterol do not develop Alzheimer's disease more often than people with low cholesterol.[23]

Furthermore, in the PROSPER and the WOSCOPS trials, the mental functions of the participants were examined regularly, but no difference was noted between the two groups at the end of the trials.

Not unexpectedly, researchers who are not employed by the pharmaceutical industry have even found negative effects from cholesterol reducing treatment. One of them is Matthew Muldoon, an American professor of internal medicine. Already after six months he noted that the memory of patients had declined.[27] Later on in my book I shall tell the reader about more serious, cerebral disturbances caused by statin treatment.

Now to the crucial question. If Alzheimer's disease is seen more often in untreated people than in people on statin treatment, is it because they have had low cholesterol for many years or is it because they have not received statin treatment? If Alzheimer's disease is seen less often in statin-treated people, is it because they have lived most of their life with high cholesterol, or is it because they have received statin treatment? Nobody knows.

Cholesterol lowering from early childhood!

Eager proponents of the cholesterol hypothesis argue for reducing cholesterol during childhood. They say that atherosclerosis starts in childhood; therefore all parents should test their children's cholesterol and teach them to eat 'properly' from the age of two. This age limit is set because the proponents, in spite of their cleverness in marketing and persuading, would have great difficulty in declaring that milk, an allegedly poisonous food item for adults, is harmful for babies as well.

Their argument for starting cholesterol lowering in childhood is that the fatty streaks, the thin layer of cholesterol-loaded cells situated on the inside of most arteries, are seen before we are born and they also claim that these fatty streaks are the precursors of atherosclerosis.

Fatty streaks are found in the vessels of all children, even in populations where atherosclerosis is rare.[28] Therefore, the mere presence of fatty streaks is not enough for producing atherosclerosis, something else is necessary. There is no evidence either that fatty streaks are due to high cholesterol, or that they disappear if we lower childrens' cholesterol. In addition, high cholesterol in childhood does not mean that cholesterol will be high later in life. Several studies have shown that about half of the children with high cholesterol at age two have a normal cholesterol when they reach puberty.[28]

If it were true that it remained high in adulthood and caused heart disease later in life, how should we treat the children? The answer from the proponents is: by diet! Certainly, many children are now eating chemically processed margarine and a variety of peculiar, synthetic nonfat products instead of the nutritious and natural foods such as milk, cheese and eggs. We can only guess at the dangers that are threatening a child by following such a regime for the rest of their life.

Furthermore, the effect of diet on blood cholesterol is hardly measurable, in particular in children. The only way to lower cholesterol effectively is by drugs; even the proponents admit that. We have no evidence, that a possible benefit from cholesterol lowering from the age of two may balance the side effects from an unhealthy diet or a daily intake of drugs during 50-60 years because luckily, such trials have never been done. Rather, a treatment of that kind may create families of unhappy hypochondriacs, obsessed with their blood chemistry and the composition of their diet.[28]

Sources

1. Ravnskov U. BMJ 1992;305:15-19.
2. Salonen JT and others. Ann N Y Acad Sci 1982;382:423-37.
    Tuomilehto J and others. BMJ 1986;293:1068-71.
3. Frick MH and others. N Engl J Med 1987;317:1237-45.
4. Hjermann I and others. Lancet 1981;2:1303.
5. Brown G and others. N Engl J Med 1990;323:1289-98.
6. Brown G and others. Circulation 1984;70:18-24.
7. Glagov S and others. N Engl J Med 1987;316:1371-5.
8. Ravnskov U. QJM 2002;95:397-403.
9. JAMA 1984;251:351-64.
10. Circulation 1973;47(suppl1)1-50.
    JAMA 1970;214:1303-13.
    JAMA 1972;220:996-1008
    JAMA 1973;226:652-7.
    JAMA 1975;31:360-81.
11. Br Heart J 1978;40:1069-1118Lancet 1980;2:379-85.
12. JAMA 1982;248:1465-77.
13. Miettinen TA and others. JAMA 1985;254:2097-102
14. Scandinavian Simvastatin Survival Study Group. Lancet 1994;344:1383-9.
15. MRC/BHF Heart Protection Study. Lancet 2002;360:7-22.
16. N Engl J Med 1998;339:1349-57
17. Sacks FM and others. N Engl J Med 1996;335:1001-9.
18. Bradford RH and others. Arch Intern Med 1991;151:43-9.
19. Shepherd J. and others. N Engl J Med 1995;333:1301-7
20. Downs JR and others.JAMA 1998;279:1615-21.
21. Ridker PM and others. N Engl J Med 2008;359:2195-2207.

22. Shepherd J and others. Lancet 2002;360:1623-30.
23. Schalk BWM and others. Age and Ageing 2004;33:266-72.
24. de Lau LML and others. Am J Epidemiol 2006;164:998-1002.
25. Mielke MM and others. Neurology 2005;64:1689-95.
26. Elias PK and others. Psychosom Med 2005;67:24-30.
27. Muldoon MF and others. Am J Med 2000;108:538-47.
28. Ravnskov U. Lancet 2000;355: 69

How to Keep A False Idea Alive

CHAPTER 7
How to Ignore Contradictory Evidence

In the streets, the garbage lies
Protected by a million flies
The roaches so big You know that they got bones
They moved in and made a tenement home

Guns N' Roses

According to the map you have reached the top of a mountain, but when you look around, you cannot see anything else but flat fields. Which is right? Your eyes or your map? Most of us would say that our eyes can't fool us that much. Some of us may check the longitude and the latitude on the map to see if they are identical with those given by the GPS. If they are, we are not in doubt, it is the map writers who have made a mistake. In the field of cholesterol research, most students have blind faith in the map. This is evidently a large mountain, they say, even if it looks like a meadow.

Helsinki Heart Study

In the previous chapter I told you about the Helsinki Heart Study,[1] a trial which is often used as an argument for cholesterol reduction. I assume that readers familiar with the cholesterol lowering trials wonder, why the trial directors experimented on healthy people only? Why didn't they try their treatment on patients with heart disease? If anyone is at risk for a heart attack it is those who already have had one.

They did indeed, but the result was miserable. After five years, seventeen of those who took the drug gemfibrozil had died from a heart attack, compared to only eight in the placebo group. The directors were eager to stress that this difference was most probably due to chance (the map can't be wrong). In the summary of their report they wrote that the number of fatal and non-fatal heart attacks did not differ significantly between the two groups.

However, among those classified as 'cardiac deaths', they had included a small number of events called 'unwitnessed deaths', meaning those where the cause of death was unknown. It is not self-evident that an unwitnessed death is due to a heart attack, and such deaths should, of course, have been classified otherwise. In fact, if they had excluded the unwitnessed deaths, most of whom belonged to the untreated control group, there were more than three times more fatal heart attacks in the treatment group. That is sixteen deaths in the treatment group versus five in the untreated group and this difference was statistically significant. The directors of the study admitted that the result was not in accord with previous experience. They had a number of explanations. As the trial was only an expedient byproduct of the original trial, the number of individuals had been too small to give reliable results. To avoid too much fuss the unsuccessful part of the trial was not published until six years later in a less prestigious and less well known medical journal.[2]

The Oslo trial

One method of obtaining benefit in a trial is to use several kinds of intervention at the same time. This is OK if the authors tell the readers what they have done, but often they forget to do that. In a report from the Oslo trial, the authors mentioned two types of intervention, diet and smoking cessation. They did not tell us that the treatment group also reduced their body weight. From the tables it appears that at the end of the trial, the mean weight difference between the two groups was about 15 lbs (6.8 kg).[3] We know that the risk of diabetes and high blood pressure is greater for overweight people, and diabetes and high blood pressure predispose to heart disease. Now to the crucial question. Which of the measures produced the decisive effect in the Oslo trial? Was it the diet, was it smoking cessation, or was it the weight loss? Nobody knows.

Whom should we cite?

Science Citation Index is an interesting aid for scientists. Here you can see how often a scientific paper has been cited by other scientists and by whom and where. It is interesting to see how often the LRC trial[4] has been cited. Remember that this trial was the one that persuaded the Americans to start the cholesterol campaign. Let us also see how many have cited the unsuccessful Miettinen trial,[5] the trial where mortality increased in the treatment group. Both papers dealt with the same subject and were published in the same journal. It follows that they should be cited equally often.

That the LRC trial, at least according to its directors, was supportive, and the Miettinen trial was not, is unimportant because the aim of research is to find the truth.

	LRC trial	Miettinen trial
First year	109	6
Second year	121	5
Third year	202	3
Fourth year	180	1

This table shows the number of citations of a cholesterol-lowering experiment with a positive outcome and of an experiment with a negative outcome during the first four years after their publication. As you see , researchers love the LRC-trial. They cite it repeatedly. Why should they mention the disturbing figures from the Finnish experiment? Don't you try to forget your own bad experiences in your private life yourself?

Meta-analysis
Certain treatments are easy to assess. The right antibiotic, for example, will cure nine out of ten women with an uncomplicated urinary infection, which means that after having treated less than fifty patients and control individuals for a few days, you will already know for certain that the drug is effective. However, before the introduction of the statins, scientists still didn't know whether cholesterol reduction was of benefit. The statisticians said that to lower mortality, many more test individuals would be necessary, probably tens of thousands.

A meta-analysis may be used to resolve the problem. In the previous chapter I told you about my own. As mentioned, the mortality from myocardial infarction was unchanged and the total mortality had increased. Also, if cholesterol lowering was beneficial, the effect should be better the more it was lowered. This was not the case.

Did the reader understand that there was no cholesterol mountain? No, No. Instead my analysis[6] provoked harsh comments. According to my critics, it was a mistake to include the trials with serious side effects and those that did not satisfy the usual scientific standards.

The result wasn't better after the exclusion of these trials, however.

Even if the benefit was trivial I had ignored the fact that high cholesterol was a risk factor for myocardial infarction. Please take a look at the map, Dr. Ravnskov!

What I also found was that all trials with a positive outcome had been cited six times more often than the trials with a negative outcome. The trial directors themselves had been especially unwilling to cite unsupportive trials, because no trial considered unsupportive by their directors had been cited in any other trial report. The reason why these positive trials were cited more often, wrote the critics, was that they were of a much better quality than the negative trials.

4S

There is no doubt that statin treatment may be of benefit for patients with heart disease. The effect is trivial, however, as I have described in a previous chapter and it has nothing to do with cholesterol.

How do I know that, you may ask. Because there is no exposure-response, meaning that the effect is the same whether you lower cholesterol just a little or by more than fifty percent. This fact has appeared from several of the trials, including the first one, 4S.[7] Nothing is mentioned about it in the trial report, but when the results were presented for the doctors in southern Sweden, the lack of exposure-response was evident judged from the data presented at the meeting. When I pointed it out, it was obvious that the speaker had not realized it himself; neither did he understand that this phenomenon is completely devastating for the cholesterol hypothesis.

Four years later a new report was published from the 4S trial, and in that paper the authors claimed that exposure-response was present.[8] The analysis concerned only the first year of the trial, however. In a letter published in Läkartidningen, the Journal of the Swedish Medical Association, I asked Anders G Olsson, one of the authors to explain why they had published the calculations for the first year only, not for the whole period. I also reminded him about the results from the whole period shown at the meeting, where he was present as well. He answered with the following words: *Anyone obsessed by a particular idea is able to draw cocksure conclusions from selected subgroup analyses.* [9]

I am still wondering to whom he referred.

Sources
1. Frick MH and others. N Engl J Med 317, 1237-45, 1987.
2. Frick MH and others. Ann Med 1993;25:41-5.

3. Hjermann I and others. Lancet 2, 1303-10, 1981. The weight loss in the treatment group is easily overlooked because body weight was not given in kilograms but in relative body weight (body weight divided by the square of body height).

4. JAMA 1984;251:351-64.

5. Miettinen TA and others. JAMA 1985;254:2097-102.

6. Ravnskov U. BMJ 1992;305:15-9.

7. Scandinavian Simvastatin Survival Study Group. Lancet 1994;344:1383-9.

8. Pedersen T and others. Circulation 1998;97:1453-60.

9. Olsson AG. Läkartidningen 1999;96:1949.

CHAPTER 8
How to Exaggerate Insignificant Results

I got a very good friend in the CIA
And he says that he never takes bribes
But he's telling lies
'Cos he's into me
He knows I wanna be
Headline hustler
Scandal maker
Headline hustler
Money taker
Gouldman/Stewart (10 CC)

A few cholesterol researchers have observed that they got lost when they followed the map. They can't see any cholesterol mountain, but isn't there a small hill? Yes, of course, and very soon they are able to explain that the map writers were not wrong at all; they just missed a few details. Here are a few examples of the way they have succeeded in converting small hills into large mountains.

The Finnish Mental Hospital Study
This is one of the most often cited trials when researchers want to tell us about the benefit of avoiding saturated fat. About 700 middle-aged male patients were studied at two mental hospitals in Finland. At one of them the patients were given a diet low in saturated fat and cholesterol and high in polyunsaturated fat; at the other one they ate the usual hospital diet. Six years later diets were reversed and the trial continued for another six years.[1] During the trial some of the patients dropped out, either because they were transferred to another institution or because they were discharged, and after the first six years the oldest patients in both groups were exchanged with younger patients. In total, less than a third of the patients completed all of this twelve-year long trial.

To distribute the risk factors evenly between the two groups is of course impossible with such a design.

Consequently there were considerably more smokers, more who had high blood pressure, and more who were treated with drugs in the control groups.

During both periods there were fewer people in the diet group who died from a heart attack and fewer who had other heart problems. However, with one exception, the differences were not statistically significant, although the authors had used a less demanding method to calculate the statistics, the one-tailed t-test. How could they know whether the number of heart attacks in the second period was a consequence of the diet the patients had eaten during the previous six years, or whether it was the result of their present diet?

Thus, this trial was neither randomised or blinded. The result could just as well have been due to differences in their blood pressure or smoking habits, or it could have been due to chance. What is not widely known is that the trial included female patients as well.[2] In that part of the trial there was no benefit at all, although the cholesterol was reduced more. In the report, published four years later (and never cited by anyone) the authors admitted that *although the results of this trial do not permit firm conclusions, they support the idea that also among female populations the serum-cholesterol-lowering diet exerts a preventive effect on CHD.*

Similar illogical statements flourish among research workers who prefer to believe the cholesterol hypothesis rather than their own results. Here is a typical example from a study named The Western Electric Study.[3] The aim of that study was to learn what kind of food patients with myocardial infarction had eaten previously. What the authors found was that the patients had not eaten more saturated fat than healthy people. Nevertheless, what they concluded was that *within the context of the total literature, however, the present observations support the conclusion that the lipid composition of the diet affects the level of serum cholesterol and the long-term risk of death from coronary heart disease.*

How are negative results able to give support? What do they mean by the total literature? Which literature? Alice in Wonderland perhaps?

MRFIT

As you will remember from the preceding chapters, the MRFIT trial failed to support the cholesterol hypothesis by one hundred percent. Usually, when a scientific experiment does not produce results supporting their hypothesis, the investigators admit it immediately, but this was not an ordinary experiment. 69

More than a decade of hard work and several hundred millions of dollars had been invested in what was the most ambitious medical experiment ever conducted. Hundreds of personnel including doctors, professors, statisticians, dieticians, psychologists and other experts had been engaged. More than fifty scientific reports had already been published, and thousands of apparently healthy men and their families had been persuaded to take part in time-consuming investigations, and to change their diet and their way of life for many years. How did the authors explain that all the work and the money had been spent in vain?

They didn't.

In the report from the trial, the authors divided the participants into smaller groups and excluded the group with the worst outcome. After that, the result seemed a little better. Almost all the other groups had a smaller number of fatal heart attacks; not all of them, but almost all. It was obvious, they wrote, that the outcome was favourable for those who had ceased smoking. This was the only intervention that seemed to have had an effect.

More realistic researchers admit that it was a failure. Their explanation is that the cholesterol was lowered by a mere two percent. This implies however that to change to a cholesterol lowering diet is ineffective, because the dietary intake of cholesterol in the treatment group had been cut by half, saturated fat intake had been decreased by more than 25 percent and they had eaten 33 percent more polyunsaturated oils than had the control individuals.

The angiographic trials
That the early angiographic trials were unsuccessful by any standards is very clear. The directors of these trials had a different opinion, however.

In the first one[5] they lowered cholesterol with a drug named cholestyramine (Atromidin®) the same drug that was used in the LRC trial. Five years later the coronary arteries had widened by a minimal fraction of a millimeter in four patients within the treatment group, but they had also become wider in four of the untreated patients. The only finding of interest was that the diameter of the arteries of those whose cholesterol was high from the beginning had been a little smaller than in those with normal cholesterol.

The directors of the trial had decided to analyze their results using the less demanding one-tailed t-test.

The National Heart, Lung, and Blood Institute had approved it because, as they claimed, *the weight of laboratory and epidemiological evidence provided assurance that the results could only go in one direction.*

The weight of laboratory and epidemiological evidence had certainly not provided any such assurance, however, because seven cholesterol-reducing trials had increased mortality instead of reducing it.

A new angiographic trial, called the Cholesterol-Lowering Athero-sclerosis Study, or CLAS, was started a little later.[6] To reduce cholesterol as much as possible, they gave two drugs at the same time; colestipol (Colestid®) and nicotinic acid. Two years later the arteries in the drug group had worsened a little but they had worsened even more in the untreated control group; therefore the result was seen as a success, but again, it didn't satisfy the usual definition of statistical significance and there was another problem. The adverse effects of nicotinic acid, the burning and itching sensations of the skin, are so unpleasant that no one was in any doubt about who was taking the drug, least of all the patients. Thus, the trial was neither single or double-blinded, which the authors had the honesty to admit. They called it selective blind, a suitable term that should be applied to most of the cholesterol lowering trials.

The trial director, David H. Blankenhorn, a professor of medicine at the University of Southern California, was excited, and called a press conference to announce their groundbreaking findings. For the first time, he said, they had shown *a strong and consistent therapy effect from cholesterol lowering at the level of coronary arteries.*

But didn't the previous trial directors say the same? Wasn't it the previous trial's strong laboratory and epidemiological evidence that allowed Blankenhorn and his co-workers to use the one-tailed t-test?

In a scientific report the authors usually discuss the results of similar studies in the past, especially if they have come up with results that are contrary to one's own. Nothing of that kind had appeared in the CLAS report. Not a word about the previous angiographic studies where the worsening of the arteries was independent of whether cholesterol went up or down. Nothing about the studies where the arteries worsened the most among those whose cholesterol levels were reduced.

Boosting the LRC trial

If all men in the USA with blood cholesterol as high as in the LRC trial received the same treatment and got the same result, it is easy to calculate that about two hundred lives would be saved per year, provided that the outcome was not merely a result of chance. However, in a letter to the editors of The Atlantic in 1990, Daniel Steinberg presented much better figures. Steinberg was the chairman of the consensus conference that started the cholesterol campaign in the USA based upon the results from the LRC trial. According to Steinberg, 100,000 lives could be saved each year. He also claimed that *this had been demonstrated in a large number of studies.*[7] Similar messages appeared in the report from the conference: *Now we have proved that it is worthwhile to lower blood cholesterol; no more trials are necessary. Now it is time for treatment.*[7]

Knowledge from clinical trials has taught us to be cautious about who should benefit from the treatment. If it has been successful for middle-aged men with extremely high cholesterol levels, then only middle-aged men with extremely high cholesterol levels should be treated until it has been proven that it is also beneficial for other categories of human beings. No such restrictions were evident in the report from the conference, however. It was suggested that almost everyone should lower their cholesterol, including those whose cholesterol was close to normal. Not only men, but also women, even though the LRC trial had not studied women and though all previous studies had shown that high cholesterol is unimportant for the female sex, despite the fact that no benefit had been seen in the few cholesterol lowering trials which included women. The only group of people not included for treatment were children but this was corrected later.

The LRC trial couldn't tell us anything about dietary treatment, because both groups had changed their diet. Neither could any of the previous trials. Regardless, the authors recommended a low-fat, low-cholesterol diet, because the results from LRC taken together with the large volume of evidence relating diet, plasma cholesterol levels and heart disease, supported the view that cholesterol reduction through dietary management would also be beneficial.

The conference was headed by Basil Rifkind, the director of the LRC trial. Rifkind also determined who would be invited to join the panel that formulated the final recommendations.[8] Consensus in Latin means accord or unanimity, but there was little accord or unanimity among the participants. For example Professor Michael Oliver from Scotland, director of the WHO trial, stressed that the trend toward an increased mortality from other causes was as strong as the trend toward a reduced mortality from heart disease. *Why explain these results away*, he asked.

Biostatistician Paul Meier opposed Rifkind's description of LRC: *To call a study conclusive which showed no difference in total mortality, and by the usual statistical criteria an entirely nonsignificant difference in coronary incidents, seems to me a substantial misuse of the term.*

There was no unanimity either about the suggested treatment. Somebody recommended a decrease in dietary cholesterol, other suggestions were a lowering of dietary fat of animal origin, or a reduction of the caloric intake, no matter how. In the summary of the report the conflict was solved by recommending all three dietary measures.

Some of the critics were cut off by the panel chair, Daniel Steinberg, who cited a lack of time, and requests to write a minority report were denied as inconsistent with the conference goal of consensus. Consequently, none of the many critical comments were included in the report from the conference. According to Thomas Moore,[9] who was present at the conference, the report was already written before the conference. Why waste money for a GPS device if we already have a perfect map?

Sources
1. Turpeinen O and others. Int J Epidemiol 1979;8:79-118
2. Miettinen M and others. Int J Epidemiol 1983;12:17-25.
3. Shekelle RB and others. N Engl J Med 1981;304:65-70.
4. JAMA 1982;248:1465-77.
5. Brensike JF and others. Circulation 1984;69:313-24.
   Levi RI and others. Circulation 1984;69:325-37.
6. Blankenhorn DH. JAMA 1987;257:3233-40.
7. The Atlantic, January 1990.
8. JAMA 1985;253:2080-86. My information from the consensus conference is taken from Thomas Moore's book "Heart Failure", Random House, NY 1989

CHAPTER 9
How to Explain Away Awkward Results

All I want is the truth, just give me some truth
I've had enough of reading things
By neurotic, psychotic pig-headed politicians
All I want is the truth, just give me some truth
No short haired-yellow bellied son of tricky dicky's
Gonna mother Hubbard,
soft soap me with just a pocketful of hope
Money for dope, money for rope
I'm sick to death of seeing things from
Tight lipped, condescending mama's little chauvinists
All I want is the truth, just give me some truth

John Lennon

For many years, prominent international experts have decided that saturated fat and high cholesterol are dangerous to health and they have encouraged doctors from all over the world to inform the population about it and to lower cholesterol by all possible methods. Nobody is in doubt. In the medical journals, the research writers repeat it incessantly and all health authorities do it, all kinds of health providers do it and the media reinforce the message. What can investigators do when their results are incompatible with what everybody 'knows' is the truth?

It is not an enviable situation, especially when the trials have not followed the planned path, because money is involved. What do you think will happen if one of the scientists who participate in a drug trial openly questions the methods used or the way the results are presented? Do you think that he will be invited as a well paid speaker to the next congress, or that his research will be paid for by the drug company in the future?

Even independent researchers may find it difficult to challenge an idea that is accepted by everyone. Colleagues may question their intellect, as may those who allocate research funds. Very few will dare to rock the boat. It is much easier to keep in stroke and shut one's eyes.

Let me now show you how questionable trial results are presented in the best possible manner, meaning the most profitable way, profitable for the doctor and the drug industry, but certainly not for the patients.

The trials

Is it wise to lower our cholesterol to avoid cardiovascular death, if the risk to die from another disease is increased instead? Would you rather prefer to die from cancer, for instance, a disease often preceded by a long period of pain and discomfort before it ends your life? Perhaps you would prefer Alzheimer's disease, where you loose your mind and your contact with friends and family while staying in a home for the debilitated? Or would you like to die little by little from slow suffocation due to a chronic lung disease?

Of course, none of us wants to die too early or too painfully, but remember that on average, the people who die from a heart attack or a stroke have lived just as long as other people. It is correct that these two diseases together kill more people than any other disease, but think about this; if it is inevitable that all of us must die eventually, is there a better way of dying?

Next question: would you lower your cholesterol to avoid a nonfatal heart attack or stroke? If you think that you would, remember that many patients recover and may live a long life with few sequels or none at all. Maybe you think it is worth the money (you have to take expensive drugs for the rest of your life), but only if the treatment is harmless.

Supporters of the cholesterol campaign tell us that cholesterol reduction is without risk because the side effects from the drugs are rare and mild, but is this true?

It is not, because the drug companies and their paid research staff are clever enough to cover up any adversity associated with cholesterol reduction, whether by dietary means or by drugs, and to exaggerate the trivial benefit. First I shall tell you about a trial performed by honest scientists, honest because they didn't explain away the bad side of the treatment.

The Dayton Trial

Forty years ago, Seymour Dayton and his team from the University of California in Los Angeles, studied the effect of a diet rich in soybean oil, at a nursing home for war veterans. Four hundred men ate the diet, another four hundred ate the usual American food, which was rich in animal fat.

Great efforts were made to keep both patients and doctors ignorant about who was treated and who was not.[1]

Seven years later, a smaller number among those who had eaten the soybean-oil diet had died from a heart attack, but more had died from other causes. For instance, seven had died from cancer in the diet group, but only two in the control group, and a year late the total number of deaths was significantly higher in the diet group. Moreover, when the researchers looked at the arteries of those who had died, they saw that atherosclerosis was most pronounced in those who had eaten the soy diet.

The authors of this well-performed trial did not explain why mortality from vascular disease had decreased but atherosclerosis itself had increased. They concluded that the effect of the trial was impressive, but it could not be used as an argument for recommending this diet for the entire population, since only old men had been studied and total mortality had not been reduced.

They could also have added that the number of heavy smokers was much larger among those who ate their usual diet. The larger number of heart attacks in the control group could have been a result of their smoking, not because their diet was unhealthy. The fact remains that the group who ate the soybean diet were more atherosclerotic and more had cancer although they smoked much less. Shouldn't those who re-commend cholesterol lowering warn us to do it by eating more soy products?

The harmless cholestyramine

Both cholestyramine and the supposedly innocent placebo taken in the control group in the LRC trial produced a number of unpleasant side effects. Two out of three of the men taking the drug had gas, heartburn, belching, bloating, abdominal pain, nausea and vomiting, and almost half of them suffered from constipation or diarrhoea. In the trial report, the authors assured the readers that these adverse effects were not serious, and that they could be neutralized by standard clinical means.

But how do you explain that almost half of the men in the control group had similar symptoms? Is it likely that so many previously healthy people also suffered from gas, heartburn, belching, bloating, abdominal pain, nausea, vomiting, constipation or diarrhoea? Isn't it more likely that the placebo drug wasn't an innocent sugar pill, but a drug with similar adverse effects as those produced by cholestyramine? By this trick you could say that the complaints in the treated group have nothing to do with the drug on trial.

According to the trial report *the side effects were treated by standard clinical means*. These words mean that most of these previously healthy individuals had to take laxatives, antacids or drugs to stop diarrhoea or to prevent nausea and vomiting.

A significant number within the treatment group were also admitted to hospital for operations or procedures involving the nervous system. As the directors were unable to explain how cholestyramine could harm the nervous system, they considered that these symptoms were coincidental.

Cholestyramine is still prescribed today, but few people know about its many adverse effects. At the time the public was reassured by the words of Daniel Steinberg, in The Atlantic: *The drugs in current use for lowering cholesterol levels have remarkably few side effects and, to my knowledge, no fatal side effects.*[2]

Similar words are used about the new cholesterol lowering drugs, the statins, taken today by millions of healthy people all over the world. How many are still healthy? Nobody knows because very few of them know that their weak and painful muscles, their bad memory, their sexual impotence and their cancer are not the consequences of old age, but may be caused by the drug which they have been prescribed by their doctor. Sad to say, that their doctor doesn't know it either, because according to the cholesterol experts the side effects are both rare and mild. Don't believe them. I shall tell you why.

The first statin trial

Few doctors and researchers have heard about EXCEL, the first statin trial. More than 8,000 healthy individuals (called 'patients' in the trial reports) received one of four different doses of lovastatin (Mevacor®) or a placebo. To report on any possible adverse effects, preliminary results were published after one year. No significant side effects were mentioned, but in the fine print the authors wrote that 0.5 percent had died in the treatment group but only 0.2 percent in the control group.[3] Today, twenty reports from that trial have been published in the medical journals. They tell us how well lovastatin is tolerated and how effective it is for reducing cholesterol, but no one has reported anything about the concluding outcome of the trial. Therefore I wrote to Merck, the producer of lovastatin and sponsor of the trial. They told me that the aim of the study was to see if the 'patients' tolerated the drug and because they did, they had stopped the trial after only one year.

What the statins do

Apart from their disinterest in mortality, it seems as if the drug producers have not understood how the statins work. The side effects from most drugs usually begin when the treatment starts. Therefore both the patient and the doctor understand that the drug is responsible. Side effects from statins occur much later because it is not the drugs themselves that are intolerable, but their effects on our cells. The statins inhibit not only the synthesis of cholesterol, but also that of other vital molecules, for instance ubiquinol. Probably you know ubiquinol better by its other name, coenzyme Q10, or Q10 for short.

Many doctors think that Q10 is a drug used by quacks, but this is in fact a vitally important molecule, synthesized and used by all cells for energy production. Additionally, it is an effective antioxidant meaning that it protects us against foreign substances that are able to damage our cells by oxidation.

Q10 is located to the mitochondria of our cells, and the mitochondrion is the cell's power plant. No energy is produced without Q10 and its importance is particularly great where energy is needed the most, in the muscle cells. Muscle complaints are also the most frequent adverse effect of statin treatment. Q10 does not disappear immediately when you start the treatment. The production falls and it takes some time before the patient feels anything. Any side effects due to lack of Q10 may therefore occur a long time after the treatment has begun.

Perhaps even worse is that the statins also inhibit the synthesis of another vital molecule named dolichol. This substance is crucial for the production of certain proteins vital for proper cell function. It is impossible to foresee the effects of too little dolichol meaning that we can expect any type of side effect from the statins. Dolichol does not disappear suddenly either, and the side effects may therefore appear gradually.

Muscular side effects

Authors of the trial reports say that less than one percent of statin users complain of muscle pain or weakness, also called myopathy, but this is, with all certainty, an underestimation. Independent Austrian researchers for instance have reported that this effect occurs in one out of four statin-treated patients who exercise regularly.[4] They also noted that seventeen out of twenty-two professional athletes with familial hypercholesterolemia treated with statins, stopped because of that particular side effect.[5] Competitive athletes are of course more sensitive than the rest of us because they are able to measure the slightest reduction of muscular strength with a rule or a stopwatch, but even mild symptoms may have a deleterious effect on old people who already have weak muscles. It is not a minor problem because the cheapest and the least risky way to prevent heart disease is regular exercise. In the long run it may counteract any possible benefit from statin treatment.

When muscles are damaged, the concentration of an enzyme called creatine kinase, or CK, becomes elevated in the blood. High CK is thus an early sign of muscle damage of both the skeletal muscles and the heart. We are told that high CK is seen in less than one percent, but high CK is defined as a value that is ten times higher than the normal upper limit at two successive determinations. Similarly, liver damage, another adverse effect, is reported only if the liver enzymes in the blood are more than three times higher than the normal upper limit, and again, only if it has been reported twice.

Do you think that the muscles are still functioning well after lifelong statin treatment and a CK value that is 'only' nine times higher than normal? Do you think that the liver is still able to perform its many important functions if the liver enzymes leaked into the blood have been twice as high as normal for decades?

The habit of recording muscle damage only if CK is elevated is also questionable. Even in people on statins with normal CK and without any symptoms, the muscle cells may have microscopic signs of damage.[6] This is what researchers found in ten of fourteen such 'patients'.[7] We can only guess how the muscle cells will look like after many years of treatment.

Rhabdomyolysis

In the rare cases, muscles are completely destroyed; a disease called rhabdomyolysis. Large amounts of myoglobin, the main muscle protein, leaves the muscles and is excreted in the urine, and if too much myoglobin arrives at the kidneys in a short time, it may lead to renal failure.

A few years after the introduction of Bayer's statin drug Baycol, fifty patients on such treatment were reported to have died from renal failure, and since then the number has doubled. The number of live patients with kidney failure must be much higher, because most of them will survive thanks to dialysis treatment or a kidney transplantation, but that number has not been given in any official report.

Heart failure

The heart is also a muscle. Therefore lack of Q10 may be harmful to the heart as well. Karl Folkers is a famous American biochemist who discovered the molecular structure of Q10. He also found that statin treatment reduced the concentration of Q10 and caused the heart's function to deteriorate, but if he gave the patients Q10, their heart recovered.[8] In accordance, many investigators have found that Q10 treatment is of benefit in patients with heart failure.[9]

Heart failure is not reported as an adverse effect in the trial reports, probably because patients with heart failure are routinely excluded from statin trials, and because heart failure may be seen as the result of the disease, not as an adverse effect of treatment. This is most likely what the practising doctor will think as well, because nothing is written on the drug labels about heart failure as a potential adverse effect.

Brain problems

As mentioned, the brain contains the highest concentration of cholesterol in your body and I have given you some examples of the cerebral consequences of having too little cholesterol, but there is much more.

The rate of cholesterol production is particularly high in the central nervous system of the fetus and the newborn, probably explaining the severe malformations and the dysfunctional brain which is seen in children with Smith-Lemli-Opitz syndrome. This is an inborn error of cholesterol metabolism that leads to extremely low cholesterol values.

Low cholesterol is also a frequent finding in criminals, in homicidal offenders, and in animals and people with violent or aggressive behavior, [10,11] and there is a strong association between depression, suicide and low cholesterol.[12] In a Swedish study, for example, the suicide rate was five times higher than normally among those with the lowest cholesterol.

Relapse in cocaine addiction is also associated with low cholesterol;[13] people with low cholesterol have reduced attention, concentration and word fluency,[14] and decreased cholesterol is associated with cognitive decline in the elderly.[15] It is therefore no surprise that statin treatment may have adverse effects on the brain.

Beatrice Golomb, a professor of medicine, at the University of California, has devoted much of her research to the adverse effects of statins and she is, today, the most knowledgeable researcher in this area. In a meticulous analysis of all known studies about low cholesterol and violence, she concluded that the association is causal and that the risk of creating violent behaviour by reducing cholesterol, should be taken into consideration.[16] She has also reported about patients on statin treatment, who suffered from severe irritability and who recovered after discontinuation of the drug.[17]

Other researchers have described patients who suffered with progressive dementia, who recovered after they had stopped their treatment.[18] Leslie Wagstaff and his team at Duke University searched the FDA's Med-Watch surveillance system for reports of statin-associated memory loss and found sixty cases. The symptoms varied between short-term memory loss and total amnesia. These symptoms usually occurred after several months and most of them disappeared after withdrawal of the drug.[19] In accordance, women with high cholesterol have a better memory than women with low cholesterol, and women whose cholesterol goes up have a better memory score than women whose cholesterol goes down.[20]

Total loss of memory or amnesia, is very rare, at least it was before the statins were introduced. In his book 'Lipitor, Thief of Memory', Duane Graveline, astronaut, aerospace medical researcher, flight surgeon and family doctor described how he became a victim of amnesia himself.[21] For several hours he didn't recognize his wife. He suspected that the cause might have been Lipitor and stopped taking it.

At the next physical Graveline was prescribed Lipitor again. Neither the NASA doctors, nor any of the many doctors or pharmacists whom he had consulted, had ever heard about this side effect, so he followed their advice.

Six weeks later it happened again; this time for twelve hours where he couldn't recall anything that had happened to him after high school. This time Graveline was convinced; the villain was Lipitor and he sent a letter about his experience to The People's Pharmacy.[22] Soon afterwards thousands of upset patients and relatives contacted him and told about a full array of similar adverse effects. Many cases have also been reported to the FDA. However, to date the agency has taken no action; they have not even issued a warning. *The subject is still being reviewed*, was their response to Graveline.

If you are on a statin drug, please read his books[23] or take a look at his website. Here he tells you about what has happened with the thousands of victims who have contacted him after the publication of his first book.

The number of statin users is huge; in the US alone, the numbers probably exceed more than twenty-million people.

It is frightening to think that pilots taking statins are still flying planes, truck drivers taking statins drive trucks, and parents and grandparents taking statins drive their children and grandchildren in cars.

On some drug labels you can read that bad memory is a rare adverse effect, but how do the drug company and their researchers know it is rare if they haven't studied it systematically? And if they have, why have the results of these studies not been published?

After having examined the trial reports, Joel M. Kaufmann, a retired professor in pharmacology from the University of Philadelphia found an explanation. Pharmaceutical companies split up one serious side effect into several minor groups to prevent their drug from not being approved. This is an established method to keep alarming adverse effects below the one percent level. Amnesia for instance can be split into confusion, memory weakness, senility, dementia and impaired cognitive function. A serious and rather common problem simply falls apart when split into small groups.

The nerves

If low cholesterol is bad for the brain, it is reasonable to assume that it is bad for the nerves as well. Nerve damage is called polyneuropathy. This is a distressing and very disturbing painful condition, which starts in the feet and legs and may spread to other parts of the body. The usual symptoms are burning and tingling sensations and even total loss of sensory appreciation. Polyneuropathy may also lead to muscular weakness and difficulty with walking.

In a study from Denmark, David Gaist and his team found that among the patients with polyneuropathy of unknown cause, 26 times more people were on a statin treatment when compared with healthy individuals. They had also noted that the risk increased with time.[24] What happens, you may ask, after lifelong treatment?

The problem is particularly serious for patients with diabetes, because even without statin treatment diabetics run a much greater risk of developing polyneuropathy than other people. In many countries doctors have been told to prescribe statin treatment to all diabetics as a matter of routine. In Sweden the district medical officers get better paid when they put more diabetics onto statin treatment. It is to be hoped that these doctors know that polyneuropathy may be a side effect, but the risk is that they will put the blame onto the patient's disease.

Impotency

The male sex hormone testosterone is produced by changing the cholesterol molecule a little. A natural question is whether a lowering of cholesterol means that the production of testosterone goes down. Curiously this is not the case, at least not in the short run.[25] However, several case reports about impotency after statin treatment have been published.

To study how often it may occur, British doctors asked their male patients about their sexual functions before statin treatment started. A few months later about a fifth of the patients had become impotent to some degree.[26]

It is worth mentioning that the study was sponsored by Pfizer. Their statin drug is called Lipitor, but they have not mentioned anything about this potential side effect on the Lipitor website. Why should they? If you fail, just take a Viagra, another of Pfizer's billion dollar-selling drugs.

Bad for the baby

To understand the effects of statin use during pregnancy, two research workers from America had reviewed 178 cases which were reported to the FDA. After having excluded spontaneous and voluntary abortions, they ended up with 52 cases. Almost half of these women's newborn babies had serious malformations of the brain or the limbs.[27]

That is not all. In Tel Aviv, researchers studied living placental (after-birth) tissue. If they added small doses of simvastatin to the culture medium, vital functions of the placental cells were inhibited. They concluded that these toxic effects may have caused the higher abortion rate and malformations seen in studies of animals given statins during pregnancy.[28] There is reason to believe that the many cases of spontaneous abortions, which were excluded by the American researchers, were also caused by the statins.

On the drug labels pregnant women are warned against statin treatment. How many people will read the fine print? Even so, about half of all pregnancies are unplanned, and chemically induced effects on the fetus occurs within the first two months of pregnancy.

Cancer and the statin trials

Statins produce cancer. This was the conclusion of University of California researchers Thomas Newman and Stephen Hulley after having analysed all the studies of statin-treated laboratory animals.[29] They asked themselves why these drugs had been approved by the FDA.

Defenders of statins pointed out that the doses used in the animal experiments were much higher than those recommended for clinical use, but as Newman and Hulley commented, it is more relevant to compare blood levels of the drug. In these experiments the levels that caused cancer in the animals were close to those seen in patients taking statin drugs. Today the levels are likely much higher as doctors are recommended to use doses up to eight times higher than previously.

In human beings it takes a much longer time to produce cancer than in rats and mice. Newman and Hulley therefore recommended that the statins should be used only for patients at very high risk for coronary disease, not for people with a long life expectancy, and healthy people with high cholesterol as their only risk factor belong to that category.

Caution should be exercised in the use of the statin drugs as there is much evidence to suggest that such treatment may lead to cancer in humans as well. If so, it is likely to show up first in people with the highest risk, for instance in old people. There are also great differences between the incubation period for different cancers. Those that appear the earliest are of course those that are the easiest to detect. The results from the statin trials are therefore disquieting.

Cancer and simvastatin
In the first two simvastatin trials, 4S and HPS, thirty more patients in the treatment group developed skin cancer. Although these figures appeared in the tables, the authors did not mention this alarming finding in the discussion or in the summary of the reports. The reason may be that the difference was not significant in each trial. However, if the numbers from both trials are added together, the difference becomes significant, meaning that it is highly unlikely that the result was due to chance.

Please note that we are not talking about malignant melanoma. The types of skin cancer reported in these trials was of another type. They are considered unimportant because they are easy to treat; nobody dies from common skin cancer today. However, a cancer is a cancer. If statin treatment or low cholesterol are able to create various types of cancer as in the animal experiments, the first type we should expect to see is, of course, skin cancer, simply because it is easy to detect at an early stage. Besides, people who get skin cancer are predisposed to develop other types of more vicious cancers later in life.[31]

The trial directors of the many statin trials that followed after the 4S and HPS trials have truthfully reported about the number of cancer cases that occurred during the treatment periods, but they have ignored the commonest one, skin cancer. This is of course convenient for the drug companies, but not for those who are prescribed a statin treatment for the rest of their life.

No significant increase of cancer was noted in the ten year follow-up of the 4S trial participants and the authors concluded that ten years of statin treatment does not induce cancer. Neither does ten years smoking tobacco.

Cancer and pravastatin

Another easily detectable malignancy is breast cancer. In the CARE trial thirteen women had developed breast cancer in the treatment group, but only one in the control group. Some of them were new cases; others were recurrences of previously treated breast cancers. The authors of the CARE report were eager to explain it away. These findings could be an anomaly, they wrote.[32] Since then, all patients who have undergone cancer treatment have been excluded from the trials. This is most curious because supporters of statin treatment claim that statins are able to prevent cancer. If they had included cancer patients, and if they were right, the result of the treatment might of course have been much better, but they chose not to.

There is more evidence that statin treatment may cause cancer. Let us take a look at the PROSPER trial again.

After three years the number of fatal heart attacks was significantly lower in the treatment group. Consequently, the trial was stopped for ethical reasons but at the same time more patients had died from cancer and therefore the total number of deaths was equal in the two groups.[33]

The authors were confident that the increased number of cancer cases was not an effect of the treatment because when they looked at the number who had died in all of the pravastatin trials taken together, no difference was seen. However, in this calculation they did not include the number of skin cancers.

What they also forgot to mention was that in the previous trials the participants were twenty-five years younger than in their own study. Cancer is primarily a disease of old age. Cancer cells are frequently found at the postmortems of old people who have died from something else. They are often dormant or they grow so slowly that they never become a problem, unless their growth is stimulated; by statin treatment for example.

However, instead of hoisting a flag of warning the authors wrote the following: *In view of available evidence, the most likely explanation is that the imbalance in cancer rates in PROSPER was a chance finding, which could in part have been driven by the recruitment of individuals with occult disease.*

If it were so, why didn't the occult cancers pop up among their untreated patients, because they were just as old? The fact is that the total number of deaths in the two groups was the same. The trial directors hadn't succeeded in prolonging life by using statin treatment, but they had an explanation: *The study was not considered to be adequately powered to detect an effect on all-cause mortality.* By these words they meant that either the trial included too few participants, or it went on for a too short time. Nevertheless, the PROSPER trial had included 1400 more patients than the 4S trial, and in that trial the total number of deaths was lowered significantly. The most likely explanation is of course that mortality from cancer increased and in this way balanced the decrease of heart mortality.

Cancer and ezetimibe

Cholesterol reduction has also been tried as a preventive measure in patients with narrowing of the aorta, the main artery of the body. In this experiment, named SEAS, cholesterol was lowered with two different drugs, simvastatin (Zocord®) and ezetimibe (Ezetrol®). Consequently, the cholesterol values plummeted and remained at about fifty percent below the initial value during the whole trial.[34] The treatment did not reduce the composite number of cardiovascular events, however, but the number of cancer cases increased with statistical significance.

In the report from the trial the authors, all of whom had received consulting and lecture fees from several drug companies, concluded that *long-term statin therapy has not been associated with an increased risk of cancer and as it was not associated with the degree of cholesterol lowering, it may have been a result of chance.* Obviously they already had forgotten that their trial had reduced cholesterol more than any other trial.

The allegation that statin treatment does not produce cancer has been presented repeatedly. It is based on a review of fourteen statin experiments, but in all of them skin cancer was excluded; neither had the authors analysed the frequency of cancer in individuals with a particularly high risk of cancer, for instance smokers and old people.[35] And why had they only included fourteen trials? Until today, at least 1230 controlled human statin experiments have been performed,[36] and other types of studies have given frightening results.

Cancer in other statin studies

Japanese researchers have studied whether patients with lymphoid cancers have been treated more often with statin drugs than patients admitted with non-cancer diseases. They found that more than thirteen percent of the cancer patients, but only seven percent in the control group were or had been on statin treatment.[37] Their study thus has demonstrated that statins may cause cancer in as little as four or five years, the mean treatment time in the cancer group. Again, just as with skin and breast cancer, lymphoid cancer is easily detectable.

In another Japanese study almost 50,000 patients were treated with low-dose simvastatin (Zocor®) for five years. The scary fact is that the number of patients who had died from cancer was three times higher among those whose cholesterol was reduced the most compared with those whose cholesterol was lowered less efficiently.[38]

How adversities become rare

The drug companies have developed a smart way to minimize the adverse effects of statin treatment. The method is called selection. To be included in a trial the participants must satisfy a long list of criteria. In most cases about half of those originally chosen for the trial have been excluded because they did not satisfy the selection criteria. All kinds of preexistent maladies or frailties disqualify a potential participant. As mentioned above, cancer is one of them, but also kidney or liver disease, heart failure, uncontrolled diabetes, hormonal dysfunction, and gastrointestinal disorders belong to that category, including statin intolerance. 'Lack of compliance' is a frequent cause of exclusion as well. What is meant by this term is not defined, but most likely it includes intolerance to the drug.

After the exclusion procedure potential participants are usually given a small dose of the drug to be tested, a procedure that leads to the exclusion of a further number of participants. Others are excluded because they do not meet the randomisation criteria, a curious argument as these criteria were used also before the test.

It is obvious that the participants in the statin trials represent a selection of unusually strong and healthy patients compared with those sitting in the waiting room of the doctor. This fact, when taken together with the unwillingness to record laboratory signs of organ dysfunction as an adverse effect, renders the figures for statin side effects as completely unreliable.

The notion that adverse effects are common is obvious. In the IDEAL trial for instance[39] cholesterol was reduced in almost 9000 patients with heart disease; half of them had taken a high dose of atorvastatin, while the other half had taken a normal dose of simvastatin. According to the trial report, more than 90 percent in each group had experienced adverse reactions to the treatment, almost half of which were serious. As nothing was mentioned about the character of the adverse effects I and two of my colleagues sent a request for more information to the editor of the journal where the trial report had appeared.[40] Here is the answer from the authors:

The numbers presented do not represent only drug-related adverse effects. In accordance with good clinical trial practice, the study protocol required that all observed and volunteered adverse effects, whether or not considered drug-related, should be recorded during the trial. This included worsening or increase in severity or frequency of preexisting conditions as well as minor and serious new signs, symptoms, or laboratory findings. In a population of middle-aged or elderly patients aged up to 80 years, it is rare that anyone does not have at least an episode of common cold or a minor musculoskeletal injury over a period of 5 years.

As common colds or minor musculo-skeletal injuries cannot be considered as serious side effects we sent a new letter. We pointed out that no previous trial had shown so many adverse effects. Therefore, we wanted to know more about the character of the symptoms and the authors' reasons for not classifying them as adverse effects to the treatment. The answer from the editor was that *your letter did not receive a high enough priority rating for publication*, but he encouraged us to contact the corresponding author of the article *although we cannot guarantee a response*.

Reporting adverse effects

You may probably wonder, why all these side effects haven't been reported to the authorities by the practising doctors. Malcolm Kendrick, a British general practitioner and a member of our association THINCS (The International Network of Cholesterol Skeptics), once explained why: *Filling in a report is a hassle in the UK; and once you have done so, you are further bombarded with questionnaires by the pharmaceutical company involved.*

Dr. Kendrick estimated that filing an adverse drug report, then dealing with the follow up paperwork, takes about two to three hours of work. Then nothing at all happens.

No letter of thanks, no update on any other reports in the area. Total silence. *If you wanted to develop a system designed to ensure that none ever reports anything, ever again, this system seems fully up to the task. Especially as, if you do not report an adverse reaction, absolutely nothing happens to you.*

Regretfully, it works. According to a questionnaire sent to all practicing doctors in Rhode Island, the serious side effects reported to the FDA during the previous year corresponded to only one percent of the numbers who are actually seen.[41] It is fortunate that many people are able to think for themselves. According to a study from Canada, the large majority of more than 140,000 elderly people, who had been prescribed a statin drug, had stopped the medication two years later.[42]

Are the cholesterol researchers blind or what?

In a previous chapter I pointed to many studies where researchers found that high cholesterol was not a risk factor for coronary heart disease. When people who die from a heart attack have, generally speaking, the same cholesterol as healthy people, why is it that the researchers do not understand that high cholesterol was not the cause? Because they can explain everything that doesn't fit. Learn, for example, how the Finnish researchers reacted when they saw that high cholesterol wasn't a risk factor in the part of the world where most people die from a heart attack.

They had followed about 1800 healthy middle-aged and elderly men for 5-6 years to see which of the many risk factors for heart disease were the best predictors. In their paper[43] they used almost all eleven pages to show and discuss the other risk factors. In the end they commented the most 'surprising' finding in this way: *The lack of the predictive power of serum LDL cholesterol may be a result of the short follow-up because LDL conceivably increases the risk of AMI* (Acute myocardial infarction) *through promotion of the progression of coronary atherosclerosis.*

But why is high cholesterol unimportant during the 5-6 years before the heart attack arrives?

The most striking aberrations appeared in two recent studies from the US. The first one came from the medical department at the University of California in LA.[44] A total of 137,000 patients from 541 hospitals in the US had been admitted because of an acute heart attack. In all of them, their cholesterol was analysed within the first 24 hours of hospital admission. To their surprise, the authors found that their cholesterol was lower than normal when compared with the average.

To be precise, their mean total cholesterol was 174 (4.46 mmol/l) and the 'bad' LDL cholesterol was also much lower than normal.

It is not possible to explain away the result by using the argument that it was a result of chance, considering that this is the largest study of the cholesterol levels of heart patients, which has ever been published.

The researchers were of course surprised. One explanation could be the well-known fact that cholesterol goes down in patients with an acute myocardial infarction, but they rejected it, because this happens first after two-three days and the reduction is only fifteen percent at most.[45]

Did the authors, three of whom were supported by up to eight drug companies, realize that they had stumbled upon something important? That high cholesterol may not be the cause of heart disease? Of course not, *take a look at the map!* What they concluded was that cholesterol must be reduced even further.

A few months later a research group from Henry Ford Heart and Vascular Institute in Detroit came up with a similar result.[46] Again, LDL-cholesterol measured within the first 24 hours of admission was lower than normal, not higher. To be precise, in half of the 500 patients LDL-cholesterol was lower than 105 (2.69 mmol/l). They thought that something had gone wrong and were convinced that those whose LDL was below 105 had a much better chance to survive than those whose LDL was higher, because this is what all of us have been told by the American Heart Association and the drug companies repeatedly.

Three years later it appeared that among those with low LDL twenty-six patients had died, but only twelve among those with high LDL. The authors considered their finding very salient. They had warned their readers against feeling a false sense of security in patients with low LDL. Although more of those with low LDL were on statin treatment, *these patients may in fact need more aggressive risk modification.*[46]

Does statin treatment prevent cancer?

As mentioned in the previous chapters several statin experiments showed that statin treatment increased the risk of cancer. There are also at least thirty studies, which have shown that people with low cholesterol run a greater risk of getting cancer compared with people with normal or high cholesterol. The statin proponents still claim however that reducing cholesterol with statins prevents cancer.

How have they succeeded with that feat, you may ask. How do they explain away the observation that low cholesterol is associated with cancer?

What they claim is that cancer cells use cholesterol when they grow and therefore cholesterol goes down. It is true that we need cholesterol to build cells, but it is unlikely that the liver should be unable to manufacture a few extra molecules of this important substance to keep the blood cholesterol unchanged.

As I mentioned in the introduction, great amounts of cholesterol are produced every day depending on how much cholesterol we eat. If we eat too little, the production increases and vice versa. The number of cholesterol molecules necessary to produce cancer cells must be trivial when compared with the large number used for keeping the blood cholesterol unchanged and for renewing the cells of the skin, the mucous membranes and all the organs of the body. What the proponents also ignore is that in at least eight studies blood cholesterol was low fifteen to thirty years before the cancer appeared.[47]

The allegation that statin treatment prevents cancer is based on studies where the authors have compared the risk of cancer for people on statin treatment and for untreated people.[48] In some of these studies no significant difference was seen and the authors concluded that statins did not produce cancer. In some of them, there were more cancers in the untreated group. Therefore, they say, statins may be useful to combat cancer.

The comparisons are flawed because, on average, untreated people have lower cholesterol than normal because today your cholesterol must be very low to prevent your doctor from prescribing statin treatment. In contrast, people on statin treatment have lived most of their life with normal or high cholesterol. Furthermore, in many of the eighteen studies the researchers had not asked whether the 'patients' really had taken their medicine. It is a relevant question because, as I mentioned above, adherence to statin treatment is low.

If cancer is seen less often among those who are on statin treatment, a relevant question is whether it is due to a few years of statin treatment or it is due to the lifelong protection because of their high cholesterol. If untreated people have cancer more often, is it due to the lack of statins or is it due to their low cholesterol? Nobody knows. The only way to learn whether statin treatment has any influence on cancer cells is to compare untreated and treated people, all of whom have had the same cholesterol level previously, as is done in the statin trials. The reader already knows what such experiments revealed.

The FAO/WHO experts do not give the show away

In chapter 2 I told you about the dietary U-turn performed by 28 experts selected by WHO and FAO but was it really a U-turn? How come that the experts still recommend a reduction of dietary saturated fat although they admitted that the evidence was both unsatisfactory and unreliable?

That was an easy task. They just added that the null results probably reflect the unreliability of the evidence on dietary fats from cohort studies. To strengthen their argument they wrote that the evidence from metabolic ward studies clearly shows that diets low in SFA reduce total cholesterol and should therefore reduce the risk of CHD. However, *the meta-analysis of results from cohort studies – albeit from a limited number of studies – showed no association between SFA intake and CHD, demonstrating their unreliability.* Thus, we cannot rely on cohort studies.

But in a postscript the experts changed their mind, because *a recent meta-analysis of eleven cohort studies have shown a significantly decreased risk of CHD death and CHD events when PUFA* (polyunsaturated fat) *replaces SFA* (saturated fat). *Therefore, the result from the pooling of observational studies, along with supportive evidence from clinical trials of lower CHD* (coronary heart disease) *risk in high P/S diets, and the effects of PUFA to lower LDL cholesterol and the total: high density lipoprotein ratio, led the Consultation to conclude there was convincing evidence of lower CHD risk when PUFA replaces SFA.*

Let me remind you about the nature of a cohort study. In such a study the researchers have not exchanged anything; they have asked healthy people about their eating habits and then followed these people for some years. Using complicated statistical methods, they claim that if these people had eaten more polyunsaturated and less saturated fat they would have lowered their risk. What all the cohort studies have shown however, is that the risk of cardiovascular disease is the same or even lower for people who gorge in saturated fat, compared with those who follow the dietary guidelines

Another question is raised. How did they get supportive evidence from clinical trials? That was easy as well. By including the Finnish Mental Hospital study of course (see chapter 8) and by excluding four experiments with nil or negative results.[49]

Smile or scream – it is up to you.

Sources

1. Dayton S and others. Circulation 1969;40(suppl. II):1-63.
   Dayton S and others. Lancet 1968;2:1060-2.
2. The Atlantic Monthly , January 1990.

3. Bradford RH and others. Arch Intern Med 1991;151:43-9.
4. Sinzinger H and others. J Cardiovasc Pharm 40, 163-71, 2002. 46
5. Sinzinger H, O'Grady J. Br J Clin Pharmacol 57: 525-8, 2004
6. Phillips PS and others. Ann Intern Med 2002;137:581-5.
7. Draeger A. and others. J Pathol 2006;210:94-102.
8. Folkers K and others. Proc Natl Acad Sci USA 1990;87:8931-4.
9. Langsjoen PH, Langsjoen AM. Biofactors 2003;18:101-11.
10. Muldoon MF and others. BMJ 1990;301:309-14.
11. Virkkunen M. Neuropsychobiology 1983;10:65-9.
    Kaplan JR and others. Psychosom Med 1991;53:634-42.
    Golomb BA and others. J Psych Res 2000;34:301-9.
    Pentürk S, Yalcin E. J Vet Med 2003;50:339-42.
12. Morgan RE and others. Lancet 1993;341:75-9.
    Lindberg G and others. BMJ 1992;305:277-9.
    Schuit AJ and others. Lancet 1993;341:827.
    Gallerani M and others. BMJ 1995;310:1632-6
    Vevera J and others. Eur Psych 2003;18:23-7.
    Atmaca M and others. Psychiatry Res 2008;158:87-91.
    Marcinko D. and others. Progr Neuro-Psychopharm Biol Psych2007;32:1936.
13. Buydens-Branchey L and others. Psychosom Med 2003;65:86-91.
14. Elias PK and others. Psychosom Med 2005;67:24-30.
15. Schalk BWM and others. Asge Ageing 2004;33:266-72
    van den Kommer TN and others. Neurol Ageing 2009;30:534-45.
16. Golomb BA. Ann Intern Med 1998;128:478-87.
17. Golomb BA and others. QJM 2004;97:229-35.
18. King DS and others. Pharmacotherapy 2003;23:1663-7.
19. Wagstaff LR and others. Pharmacotherapy. 2003;23:871-80.
20. Henderson VW and others. J Neurol Neurosurg Psych 2003;74:1530-4.
21. Graveline D. Lipitor, thief of memory. Infinity Publishing Co. Haverford USA 2004.
22. http://tinyurl.se/abq22u
23. Graveline D. Statin drugs side effects and the misguided was on cholesterol. Duane Graveline, Merritt Island, Fl., USA 2005.
24. Gaist D and others. Neurology 2002;58:1333-7.
25. Mastroberardino G and others. J Int Med Res 1989;17:388-94
    Dobs AS and others. Metabolism. 2000;49:115-21.
26. Solomon H and others. Int J Clin Pract. 2006;60:141-5.
27. Edison RJ, Muenke M. N Engl J Med 2004;350:1579-82.
28. Kenis I and others. Hum Reprod. 2005;20:2866-72.
29. Newman TB, Hulley SB. JAMA 1996;275:55-60.
30. Scandinavian Simvastatin Survival Study Group.Lancet 1994;344:1383-9.
    MRC/BHF Heart Protection Study. Lancet 2002;360:7-22.
31. Rosenberg CA . Cancer 2006;106:654-63.
32. Sacks FM and others. N Engl J Med 1996;335:1001-9.
33. Shepherd J and others. Lancet 2002;360:1623-30.
34. Rossebö AB and others. N Engl J Med 2008:359:1343-56.
35. Cholesterol Treatment Trialists Collaborators. Lancet 2005;366:1267-78.

36. Brugts JJ and others. BMJ 2009;338:b2376doi:10.1136/bmj.b2376
37. Iwata H and others. Cancer Sci. 2006;97:133-8.
38. Matsuzaki M an others. Circ J 2002;66:1087-95 .
39. Pedersen TR and others. JAMA 2005;294:2437-45.
40. Ravnskov U and others. JAMA 2006;295:2476.
41. Scott HD and others. Rh I Med J 1987;70:311-6.
42. Jackevicius CA and others. JAMA 2002;288: 462-7.
43. Salonen JT and others. Circulation 1991;84:129-39.
44. Sachdeva A and others. Am Heart J 2009;157:111-7.
45. Gore JM. Am J Cardiol 1984;54:722-5.
    Sewdarsen M and others. Postgrad Med J 1988;64;352-6.
46. Al-Mallah MH. Cardiol J 2009;16:227-33.
47. Williams RR and others.JAMA 1981;245:247-52
    Keys A and others. Am J Epidemiol 1985;121:870-83
    Salmond CE and others. BMJ 1985;290:422-4.
    Törnberg SA and others. J Natl Cancer Inst 1989;81:1917-21
    Kreger BE and others. Cancer 1992;70:1038-43
    Sachet AJ and others. Am J Epidemiol 1993;137:966-76
    Chang AK and others.Prev Med 1995;24:557-62
    Eichholzer M and others. Am J Clin Nutr 2000;71:569-74.
48. Jackevicius CA and others. JAMA 2002;288:462-7.
49. Research Committee. Lancet 1968;2:693-700.
    Woodhill JM and others. Adv Exp Med Biol 1978;109:317-30.
    Burr ML and others. Lancet 1989;2:757-61.
    Frantz ID and others. Arteriosclerosis 1989;9:129-35.

CHAPTER 10
How To Lie Convincingly

There's room at the top they're telling you still
But first you must learn how to smile as you kill
If you want to be like the folks on the hill
John Lennon

This is a provocative title for a chapter in a serious book, but how else should I characterize experienced researchers' deliberate exclusion of facts that do not fit their pet hypothesis? What about their allegation that a clinical research study has shown this or that, when it hasn't? Let me start with Ancel Keys, the inventor of the diet-heart idea.

As I told you in chapter 2 Keys convinced a whole world of medical scientists that fat food was the culprit.[1] But why did Keys present data from six countries only? At that particular time the information was available from twenty-two. This is what two American scientists revealed four years later.[2] Their conclusion was clear: *The apparent association is greatly reduced when tested on all countries for which data are available instead of the six countries used by another investigator.* The death rate from coronary heart disease in Finland, for instance, was seven times that of Mexico, although fat consumption in the two nations was almost the same.

Another allegation by Keys was that cholesterol goes up the more fat we eat. In one of his papers he had illustrated his idea with a graph showing the relationship between the total amount of fat in the food and the mean cholesterol level in eighteen populations.[3] It was possible to draw a straight line through almost all of the points, which Keys had selected. This is an amazing result considering the uncertainties associated with such data. Keys did not say from where he had collected them and the reader is therefore unable to check if they are correct.

It is easy to find populations that do not fit with Keys' beautiful diagram. Suffice it to mention the Masai people, but there are many more. Nobody has been able to confirm Keys' findings either.

In his later study named Seven Countries, he claimed that the association was far better between cholesterol and the intake of saturated fat. How could it be better? The answer is that in the Seven Countries study there was no association at all between cholesterol and the total fat intake.

Readers who want to know how Keys explained the discrepancy between his two studies will search in vain.

The odd Framingham results

Let me return to the observation that high cholesterol was not a risk factor after age forty-seven and that mortality increased among those whose cholesterol went down.[4] Did the Framingham researchers question their own findings? Did they tell people that the map writers were wrong; that high cholesterol wasn't anything of which to be afraid?

Not at all. Instead you can read the following in a statement from the American Heart Association and the National Heart, Lung, and Blood Institute: *The results of the Framingham study indicate that a 1% reduction…of cholesterol corresponds to a 2% reduction in CHD risk.*[5]

No, it isn't a printing error, and this statement has been published repeatedly in numerous scientific reports, although according to the original report mortality increased by 11 %.

Two years later the Framingham researchers published a new report concerning the same thirty years of follow-up. Without presenting anything other than complicated ratios and statistical calculations, and without referring to their previous report, they stated: *The most important overall finding is the emergence of the total cholesterol concentration as a risk factor for CHD in the elderly.*[6]

Scott Grundy

In 1992 the American science journalist Gary Taubes published an article entitled 'The Soft Science of Dietary Fat' in the prestigious Science Magazine. He had examined the scientific basis for the dietary advice on fat and concluded that the vilification of saturated fat was not based on science, but was the result of political maneuvers.[7]

Scott Grundy, an American professor in internal medicine, is one of the most influential advocates for the cholesterol campaign. He has chaired a number of American Heart Association committees including the Adult Treatment Panel of the National Cholesterol Education Program. He is also the editor in chief of International Atherosclerosis Society. After the publication of Taubes' article he sent a letter to Science Magazine in protest. Here are some quotations from his letter:

The significance of saturated fatty acids has been demonstrated by an enormous number of high-quality studies carried out with dietary fat in the fields of animal research, epidemiology, metabolism and clinical trials.... Several trials reveal that substitution of unsaturated fatty acids for saturated fatty acids lowers the incidence of CHD....Evidence is abundant that elevated LDL is a major cause of CHD and that lowering serum LDL levels reduces CHD risk.[8]

Anyone familiar with the scientific literature in this area knows that nothing could be further from the truth. Together with some colleagues I sent a letter to the editor in which we pointed out that none of Grundy's references had supported his statements, some of them were even contradictory.[9]

Needless to mention that Grundy did not respond. He followed one of the main rules of the cholesterol campaign: Ignore the critics! Why didn't other researchers react? If a young researcher had made the same mistake, his career would have ended abruptly but if you have reached a sufficiently high position in the medical hierarchy, you are obviously safe.

'Diet and Health'

The largest and most influential review of the scientific literature, the very foundation of the campaign, was written by scientists at the National Institutes of Health and entitled 'Diet and Health'.[10]

A scientific review is, just like this book, a comprehensive analysis of all papers published about a specific issue. Reviews spare much work for other colleagues provided that they are complete and correct, and reviews written by distinguished scientific bodies are supposed to meet such standards.

When I started my cholesterol research I was curious to know why cholesterol is bad if it is carried by LDL. Let us take a look at the arguments presented in 'Diet and Health'.

The authors started with the following statement: *LDL has the strongest and most consistent relationship to individual and population risk of CHD, and LDL-cholesterol is centrally and causally important in the pathogenetic chain leading to atherosclerosis and CHD.*

Obviously not a good starter. At that time very few papers had given the result of LDL analyses. For example, in the hundreds of reports from the Framingham project, almost nothing was mentioned about LDL cholesterol. Where was the evidence for that statement?

The authors referred to four publications. 99

The first two gave no support,[11,12] and the third did not mention LDL-cholesterol at all.[13] The fourth was the National Cholesterol Education Program, but this was, just as Diet and Health, another large review without original data.[14] One of the conclusions here was that *a large body of epidemiological evidence supports a direct relationship between the level of serum total and LDL-cholesterol and the rate of CHD.*

According to the authors the large body of epidemiological evidence consisted of three papers. In the first one I was unable to find anything about LDL cholesterol;[15] the second paper gave no support,[16] and the third was yet another review. Here, almost nothing was written about LDL-cholesterol except for the following: *Longitudinal studies within populations show a consistent rise in the risk of CHD in relation to serum total cholesterol and LDL-cholesterol at least until late middle-age.*[17]

A little more cautious conclusion than in Diet and Health, but even for this statement the evidence was weak. References to six studies were given. In two of them LDL cholesterol was not analyzed or mentioned at all.[18] Two papers did not say anything about LDL cholesterol as a risk factor.[19] In the fifth report LDL cholesterol was *not* a risk factor.[20] and in the last one high LDL cholesterol was only a risk factor for men between age 35 and 49 and for women between age 40 and 44.[21]

Another conclusion in the National Cholesterol Education Program was that *the issue of whether lowering LDL-cholesterol levels by dietary and drug interventions can reduce the incidence of CHD has been addressed in more than a dozen randomized clinical trials.* During that time, only four such trials had included an analysis of LDL-cholesterol, and only in one of them was the number of heart attacks lowered significantly, and only for the non-fatal ones.[22]

Thus, the *large body of evidence* was one single study, which indeed showed that LDL-cholesterol was a risk factor, but only within a restricted age range. A correct conclusion from Diet and Health is that LDL cholesterol has *not* the strongest and most consistent relationship to individual and population risk of CHD, it is *not* centrally and causally important, and its lowering has *not* reduced the incidence of CHD in more than a dozen randomized clinical trials.

The screenees of MRFIT

The result from the MRFIT trial was a great disappointment, but this trial is still used as a strong argument, not for cholesterol lowering, but for the idea that high cholesterol causes myocardial infarction.

The argument is based on a follow-up study of the participants and it included not only the 12,000 men, who were selected for the trial, but also the more than 300,000 men who were excluded because they did not satisfy the trial criteria, the so-called screenees. The results from these two groups together have been published in 34 more or less identical papers in various medical journals, and they are cited again and again as the strongest possible proof that there is a direct association between blood cholesterol and the risk of future heart disease.

Lars Werkö, a Swedish professor in medicine and one of those who questioned the cholesterol campaign from the very beginning, asked himself whether it really was necessary to publish all of these reports thirty-four times because their results were so similar. According to Werkö the authors were obviously more interested in the mathematical treatment of large figures than in the quality of these figures or how they had been obtained.[23]

Worse than being repetitive, the data were inconsistent and highly questionable. For instance, the number of screenees varied greatly between the studies, from 316,099 to 361,266. In particular, Werkö questioned the reports, the authors of which had given the cause of death of all the participants, because it is highly unlikely, not to say impossible, that all of 361,266 men could have been tracked after all these years.

During the initial screening it had been discovered that in one of the reports the authors had falsely increased the number of participants, probably to obtain more research money from the NIH. This embarrassing matter received little attention, however. In spite of all these irregularities, MRFIT is still cited as *the most exact database regarding the relation of risk factors to mortality in the healthy male US population.*

Authoritative misleading

In 2007 British researchers published a review of 61 studies the authors of which had followed about 900,000 healthy individuals for several years.[24] The aim was to see whether people´s blood cholesterol was able to predict their risk of dying from a heart attack. The authors concluded that high cholesterol was associated with heart mortality in all ages and in both sexes, but not with stroke. They were of course concerned about the latter, but as the statin trials had lowered the risk of stroke they wrote that irrespective of their findings *such treatment should be guided principally by the definite evidence from randomised trials.*

I was of course curious to know how they had reached to these results because as mentioned in chapter 4 most studies have shown that high cholesterol is not a risk factor for old people and many studies have shown that old people with high cholesterol live the longest.

By examining the report I found that they had ignored at least eleven studies.[25-35] In one of them high cholesterol was a risk factor, but only for men below age 49.[34] In another study high cholesterol was a risk factor, but so was low cholesterol as well.[29] In the rest, high cholesterol was not a risk factor at all. Why had they excluded all these studies and were there other inaccuracies?

By examining each study I found that the number of participants given in the British review were not in accord with the figures given in the original reports. Just to mention that in one of them[36] the review said 9603 participants, but the original report said 37,891; in another one the review said 1783 participants, but according to the original report there were 5749,[37] and one of the studies did not mention cholesterol at all.[38]

Obviously the authors had thought that nobody would care to check the data in a complicated review originating from a highly respected university and produced by more than 100 scientists from all over the world.

Plant sterols

Cholesterol is an important constituent of plants as well, although the molecule looks a little different. There are several types of plant cholesterol; together they are named plant sterols. A typical Western diet contains 400-500 mg plant sterols, but little is taken up in the gut. Human and plant cholesterol compete for uptake in the gut. If you eat much plant sterol, your intake of normal cholesterol goes down. This fact got Unilever the idea to add plant sterols to their food products; in the first hand to margarine. The product is named 'Promise activ' in the US, and 'Flora pro-activ' or 'Becel pro.activ' in other countries.

It is correct that cholesterol goes down if we eat much plant sterol, but that doesn't mean that it is able to prevent heart disease, because no one has ever tested that in a scientific experiment. What happens is that our own cholesterol is exchanged with a foreign type of cholesterol, not only in the blood but also in our cells and cell membranes.

Is this really a good idea? Isn't it likely that the molecular differences between animal and plant sterols have a meaning? I think so, and science is in support of my view.

Several studies have shown that even a mild elevation of plant sterols in the blood is a risk factor for heart disease,[39] and the findings in people with a rare inborn disease named sitosterolemia are in accord.

These people absorb much more plant sterols than normally and all of them develop atherosclerosis early in life.

Statin treatment lowers blood cholesterol, but at the same time it raises the level of plant sterols. In the 4S-trial about 25% of the patients had a mildly elevated level of plant sterols before treatment. In this group statin treatment resulted in a further increase of plant sterols and the number of heart attacks was twice as high compared with the patients with the lowest plant sterol levels. This means that for about 25% of the many millions of people on statin treatment, their risk of heart disease may increase, not decrease.

In spite of that, Unilever still advertise their margarine and other food products with high contents of plant sterols: *Enjoy heart healthy buttery spread with Promise!*

And there is much more

The above are just a few examples of deliberately misleadings. The scientific literature about fat, cholesterol and heart disease is riddled with false statements. Most of them are written by credulous scientists who cite the official reviews in good faith; others come from authors who must know better.

In 1995 I published a paper entitled 'Quotation bias in reviews of the diet-heart idea' in which I presented a large number of intentional mis-quotations and statements.[40] The sad story is that nobody reacted.

Sources

1. Keys A. J Mount Sinai Hosp 1953;20:118-39.
2. Yerushalmy J, Hilleboe HE. NY State J Med 1957;57:2343-54.
3. Keys A and others. Ann Intern Med 1958;48:83-94.
4. Anderson KM and others. JAMA 1987;257:2176-80
5. Gotto AM and others. Circulation 1990; 81:1721-33
6. Castelli WP and others. Am J Cardiol 1989;63:12H-19H
7. Taubes G. Nutrition. Science 292, 2536-2545, 2001.
8. Grundy SM. Science 293, 801-4, 2001.
9. Ravnskov U and others. Science 295, 1464-5, 2002.
10. National Research Council. Diet and Health. National Academy Press, Washington, DC, 1989.
11. Medalie JH and others. J Chron Dis 1973;26:329-49.
12. Gordon T and others. Am J Med 1977;62:707-14.
13. Watkins LO. Am J Cardiol 1987;57:538-45
14. The Expert Panel. Arch Intern Med 1988;148:36-69.
15. Grundy SM. JAMA 1986;256:2849-56.
16. Hulley SM, Rhoads GG. Metabolism 1982;31:773-7.
17. Kannell WB and others. Circulation 1984;70:157A-205A

18. Yaari and others. Lancet 198 ;1:1011-5.
    Keys A. Seven Countries. Harvard University Press, 1980
19. Rhoads CG and others. N Engl J Med 1976;294:293-8.
    The Pooling Project Research Group. J Chron Dis 1978;31:201-306.
20. Prevent Med 1979;8:612-78.
21. Kannell and others Ann Intern Med 1979;90;85-91.
22. The Multiple Risk Factor Intervention Trial, the Newcastle Trial, the Lipid Research Clinics Trial, and the Helsinki Heart Study.
23. Werkö L. J Intern Med 1995;237: 507-518.
24. Prospective Studies Collaboration. Lancet 2007;370:1829-39
25. Siegel D et al. Am J Epidemiol 1987;126:385-99.
26. Dagenais GR et al. Can J Cardiol 1990;6:59-65.
27. Rubin SM et al. Ann Intern Med 1990;113:916-20
28. Bass KM et al. Arch Intern Med 1993;153:2209-16
29. Shestov DB et al. Circulation 1993;88:846-53
30. Corti MC et al. JAMA 1995;274:539-44.
31. Simons LA et al. Atherosclerosis. 1995;117:107-18.
32. Weverling-Rijnsburger AW et al. Lancet. 1997;350:1119-23.
33. Daviglus ML et al. JAMA 2004;292:1588-92
34. Ulmer H et al. J Womens Health 2004;13:41-53
35. Pearte CA et al. Circulation 2006;113:2177-85
36. Reunanen A and others. Acta Med Scand 1983;673(suppl):1-120.
37. Caerphilly Collaborative Group. J Epidem Community Health 1984;38:259-62.
38. Shaper AG and others. BMJ 1981;283:179-86.
39. Weingärtner O and others. Eur Heart J 2009;30:404-9
40. Ravnskov U. J Clin Epidemiol 1995;48:713-719.

CHAPTER 11
How To Ignore Alternative Explanations

You know that life is short and talk is cheap
Don't make promises that you can't keep
If you don't like the song I'm singing, just grin and bear it
All I can say is if the shoe fits wear it
If you must keep talking please can you make it rhyme
'cause your mind is on vacation
and your mouth is working overtime
Van Morrison

Medical science is based on observations and experiments on living creatures. Very often the results from such activities can be interpreted in several ways and to go further and become wiser, more studies are necessary. For true scientists the main purpose is to see if the findings accord with the prevailing hypothesis. Does it fit with what we can observe in the real world? Is the outcome of an experiment what we should expect if the hypothesis is true?

This type of research is named falsification. If new well-designed and well-performed investigations contradict our hypothesis, it has been falsified. In this situation scientists should reject it and try to find another one that fits better with the available evidence.

Less scrupulous scientists are tempted to choose another way, in particular if the results run counter to established wisdom. It is much easier to ignore contradictory findings or to try to interpret them in a way so they seem to fit. Their colleagues become satisfied and it is much more profitable. It is particularly so when it comes to the current wisdom about atherosclerosis and heart disease, because the cholesterol hypothesis is a gold mine for the food and drug industries and as long as you stick to it they will support you money-wise in many different ways.

Much saturated fat and low cholesterol?

The allegation that cholesterol goes up if we eat too much saturated fat should have been abandoned by all scientists, when their colleagues returned from Africa. How is it possible to maintain that idea, when it appeared that individuals with the lowest cholesterol ever measured in healthy people ate more than twice as much saturated fat than most of us do?

The usual argument is that the Masai people's metabolism or lifestyle must be different from our own. For instance, in one of his papers Ancel Keys stated that ... *the peculiarities of those primitive nomads have no relevance to diet-cholesterol-coronary heart disease relationships in other populations.*[1]

According to Bruce Taylor, one of Ancel Keys' colleagues, the observations from these African tribes are not contradictory, because their ability to keep their cholesterol low is superior to other people's: As the Masai people have been isolated from other tribes for many thousands of years, they have developed this ability so well, that it has been built into their genes. [2]

Taylor's interpretation is pure nonsense. An inborn metabolic trait is either present in the genes, or it arises by mutation. If it is important for survival, the number of individuals with this property increases over time, and eventually they may outnumber those without it. However, a genetic trait that protects against a disease, which kills long after sexual maturity, has no influence, because those without that trait have already transferred their 'defective' genes to their children.

The Masai people are not an isolated tribe either. They are a warlike people who have taken cattle and women from their neighbours for thousands of years. In this way they have achieved a steady genetic renewal in their cattle and in themselves.

A relevant question is why Taylor didn't study Masai people with a more normal intake of saturated fat? If he was right, their cholesterol should be even lower. He could for instance have studied Masai people who had moved to Nairobi, as did José Day, a more open-minded British researcher. What Day found was that although their intake of saturated fat was much less extreme, their cholesterol was twenty-five percent higher.[3]

Monkey tricks

Taylor is also known because he is cited for having produced the first heart attack in a monkey fed with large quantities of cholesterol.[4]

Together with his colleagues he studied wild rhesus monkeys kept individually in small dog cages. The monkeys hated their food, ate only a little, threw the rest and went on hunger strikes. It wasn't easy to take blood from the monkeys either; they resisted violently and screamed, urinated and defecated.

After four years one of them had a heart attack. The scientist found it interesting that this animal was particularly nervous, but they didn't tell the reader why it was interesting. Obviously they didn't know that mental stress is a strong risk factor for heart disease and that stress also raises cholesterol. They were convinced that the cholesterol-rich fodder was to blame.

Less saturated fat but more heart disease

The Japanese migrant study is well-known and is often use as an argument for avoiding saturated fat. When that study was performed the Japanese people ate little animal fat, their cholesterol was low, and heart disease was rare. It is tempting to link these facts with the results from the migrant study in hand. What the investigators found was that when Japanese people emigrated to the US, their cholesterol went up and they died more often from myocardial infarction and, during this time, American food was rich in saturated fat. Isn't this a wonderful demonstration of the importance of avoiding saturated fat?

One of the researchers was Michael Marmot, who has taught us much about the influence of stress and social factors on heart disease. Marmot found that it was not the food that raised the emigrants' cholesterol, nor was it the higher cholesterol that increased their risk of heart disease. He could state that with certainty, because emigrants who lived together and maintained their cultural traditions kept their low risk of heart attacks, although their cholesterol had increased as much as in those who adopted a Western lifestyle.

The most striking of Marmot's findings was that emigrants who stuck with the Japanese traditions, but preferred the fat-rich American food, ran a smaller risk of myocardial infarction than those who became accustomed to living the American way of life but ate the lean, Japanese food.[5] Isn't this a wonderful demonstration of the unimportance of avoiding saturated fat?

The North Karelia project

As you recall, heart mortality decreased a little after the start of the cholesterol campaign in North Karelia.

The cause, said the Finnish researchers, was the many health-promoting measures which they had introduced. However, the mortality had fallen in the rest of Finland as well, and the decrease in mortality in North Karelia had started seven years before the start of the campaign. The Finnish investigators didn't look at the real world, however; they were confident that their map was right. Therefore they started similar campaigns in the rest of Finland.

A crucial question remains unanswered. How was it possible that heart mortality in Finland, particularly in North Karelia, increased year by year after World War II up to the 1960s? Why did North Karelia have the highest heart mortality and the highest cholesterol in the world at that particular time?

It is tempting to assume that the two facts were causally inter-connected, but why didn't the Finnish researchers consider another explanation? Had they forgotten their own history? Before World War II Karelia was a large district in Finland that stretched from the coast of the White Sea to the Gulf of Finland. Then most of Ladoga, the largest lake in Europe belonged to Finland. In 1939, three months after Hitler's invasion of Poland, the Soviet Union attacked Finland. When the Winter War ended in 1941 most of Karelia had become a province of Russia. A large part of its population was relocated within Finland; the rest disappeared into the Soviet Union. Finland had lost its second biggest city Viipuri, its industrial heartland and Ladoga, and an eighth of Finland's citizens were made refugees without the possibility of return. Many of them were now settled in North Karelia, a small part of Karelia that still belonged to Finland.

Can you imagine the sorrow and bitterness in Finland when an eighth of its population had lost everything, including some of their family members, and lived as refugees? In addition, unemployment became a serious problem in North Karelia at that time. Didn't the Finnish researchers know that mental stress is the most effective way to raise cholesterol? Didn't they know that stress is a well known risk factor for coronary heart disease?

Sources

1. Keys A. Atherosclerosis 1975;22:149-92.
2. Biss K and others. Path Microbiol 1970;35:198-204
   Ho K-J and others. Arch Pathol 1971;91:387-410.
   Biss K and others. N Engl J Med 1971;284:694-9.
   Biss K and others. Afr J Med Sci 1971;2:249-57.
3. Day J and others. Atherosclerosis 1976;3:357-61.

4. Taylor CB and others. Arch Pathol 1962;74:16-34.
   Taylor CB and others. Arch Pathol 1963;76:404-12.
5. Marmot MG, Syme SL. Am J Epidemiol 1976;104:225-47.
   Marmot MG and others. Am J Epidemiol 1975;102:514-25.

CHAPTER 12
How to Ignore The Critics

Pity Cassandra that no one believed you
But then again you were lost from the start
Now we must suffer and sell our secrets
Bargain, playing smart, aching in our hearts
Sorry Cassandra I misunderstood
Now the last day is dawning
Some of us wanted but none of us would
Listen to words of warning

Björn Ulväus, Benny Andersson

The reluctant medical journals

Usually, editors of medical journals and members of their editorial board are only experts in their own field. When they receive a manuscript about another issue, they send it to one or more colleagues who are familiar with the subject (called referees) unless it is obvious that the report is too poorly written or researched for publication. These rules, also called the Peer Review System, are created to guarantee the quality of published papers. Somebody has referred to editorial board members and their external referees as the 'gatekeepers of science'.

Referees are usually anonymous. It is therefore impossible to know whether they are qualified to evaluate the paper. Researchers compete for priority in science, for recognition and for financial support, as well as a position of status within the medical hierarchy. They may be tempted to use the referee process to hamper the work of scientists whose opinions or results they dislike and even to steal their ideas. The same is also possible for the members of the editorial board. The risk that irrelevant motives may influence the decision whether to publish a manuscript is great, especially when its authors are questioning conventional wisdom. In the following section, I shall give a few examples from my own experience.

Don't question!

When Landé and Sperry's finding was confirmed again by electron beam tomography (see Chapter 5),[1] I sent a short letter to the journal. I pointed to the many studies of dead people, which had shown the same phenomenon (the lack of an association between blood cholesterol and the degree of atherosclerosis) and I asked why the authors didn't question that atherosclerosis was caused by high LDL-cholesterol. If those with the lowest LDL-cholesterol were just as atherosclerotic as those with the highest, it seemed difficult to maintain that idea. The editor answered that *because of space limitations we are able to publish only a few letters addressing controversial issues.*

Criticism is inappropriate

In a previous chapter, I mentioned a paper of mine entitled, 'Quotation bias in reviews of the diet-heart idea'.[2] In that paper I demonstrated the many errors and false statements presented in three major reviews of the cholesterol hypothesis written by highly esteemed American experts. Before it was published in the Journal of Clinical Epidemiology it was rejected by editors of five other journals. Here are some of their objections.

First, it was inappropriate of me to criticize Diet and Health because only part of it (70 pages!) was devoted to the subject. I was asked if any of the reviews were misrepresented, through inflation or misstatement, original work cited. My answer was of course a yes; this was the conclusion of the paper.

My argument that the Framingham Study found an eleven percent increase instead of a two percent decrease of mortality for each percentage drop of blood cholesterol was *absurd*. Obviously the referee had not checked if my allegation was correct.

One of the referees asked for objective criteria for deciding whether quotations were correct, inflated, irrelevant or contradictory. I couldn't resist asking him, *What are your objective criteria for deciding whether an apple is green and not red?*

I was also blamed for not having reviewed the weight of supporting evidence. However, as I pointed out, the aim of my study was not to review the weight of evidence, but to study how unsupportive evidence was quoted.

Cancer is unimportant

There is much evidence that reducing cholesterol may produce cancer. When I saw that the number of skin cancers in the first two simvastatin trials, when taken together, was significantly higher in the treatment groups, I sent a letter to the editor of The Lancet, where both trial reports had been published. She answered that the editorial board had decided not to publish it, but to send it to the authors of the two trials, instead.

The authors never answered me, of course. I assume that my letter inspired future trial directors and the medical companies to stop reporting the number of skin cancers; because since then, this piece of information has been absent in all trial reports.

A few weeks later The Lancet published the report from the PROSPER trial where fewer died from a heart attack, but more from cancer. Again I sent a comment to the editor, where I aired my concern for the widespread practice of prescribing a drug able to produce cancer, to hundreds of millions of people all over the world and for the rest of their lives. The editor did not find my letter to be of sufficient interest, however.

A result of chance

At the same time Anders G. Olsson, a Swedish professor in cardiology with financial links to many drug companies, wrote enthusiastically in Läkartidningen about a new statin experiment, the TNT trial.[3,4] It included 10,000 patients, half of whom were given a normal dose of atorvastatin (Lipitor®) and the other half an eight times higher dose. Both Olsson and the trial directors concluded that now, finally it has been proven that cholesterol should be reduced as much as possible.

In my comment[5] I pointed out that only the number of non-fatal heart attacks had been reduced; the number of fatal cases was equal in both groups, or to be more correct, a few more had died in the high-dose group. Olsson answered that the trial had been too small (!) to determine whether mortality had been influenced; the finding was therefore a result of chance.[6]

Another curious fact was that the authors had gained access to the data less than six weeks before it was published. How had it been possible within such short time to check all the data from such a gigantic trial, to perform the relevant statistical calculations, to write the eleven page report, to get it accepted by the many coauthors, and to get it reviewed by the referees and the editorial staff?

Wasn't it more likely that the authors had been sent a report produced and written by outside experts who were paid by the drug company, so-called ghostwriters?

Olsson answered that he had asked the main author John LaRosa how they had handled the reporting. According to LaRosa three of the authors had written the report and all of them were experienced frontline researchers. Olsson had been a coauthor of large trials himself and he could tell me how anxious they had been to present important observations for the benefit of the patients and the general public as soon as possible.

Exposure-response is unimportant

In 2002 I published a systematic review of the many previous angiographic trial reports.[7] My main finding was that none of them had found a relationship between the degree of cholesterol lowering and the angiographic changes, meaning that the plaques or the diameter of the arteries increased or decreased haphazardly whether cholesterol was reduced a lot or not at all. This finding, the lack of exposure-response, is of course incompatible with the idea that high cholesterol is the cause of atherosclerosis.

During the preceding three years I had sent the manuscript to the editors of six other medical journals, all of whom rejected it. In most cases the paper was discarded directly without letting any external experts evaluate it. Two of the journals sent it to referees; all of them rejected it with irrelevant arguments. Here are some of their objections.

This review is based on the statement that lack of exposure–response indicates lack of causality. This may be true in some cases, but not for the majority...

Even if atherosclerosis growth is causally related to LDL-cholesterol concentrations, reductions of LDL cholesterol need not necessarily lead to reductions of atherosclerosis growth...

It is unclear whether the lack of an exposure-response relationship at the level of the coronary arteries can be extrapolated to atherosclerosis of the entire vascular system...

If atherosclerosis is caused by high cholesterol, its reduction should of course be of benefit; this is the very meaning of causality. It is also highly unlikely that the cause of atherosclerosis is another one in other parts of the vascular system.

There were many more objections from the referees, but they were just as irrelevant.

Nothing new

In several of my papers I have questioned the allegation that saturated fat is dangerous to health. My largest and most comprehensive review has hitherto been rejected by the editors of nine medical journals, most often without referee assistance. Common arguments were *lack of space* or *the evidence presented is not convincing*, or *this has been said before*. The Journal of Internal Medicine rejected it because *the manuscripts have to be evaluated primarily on novelty and priority*, and the editor sent me the comments from one of the reviewers. Here are some of them.

I think this could be a good discussion piece but unfortunately the author has quoted only selectively and used only evidence that suits his purpose and ignored evidence that didn't fit, which he accuses the proponents of saturated fat of doing...

Cohort studies such as HU 1997 from the Nurses study which show a clear relationship are not quoted.

The question is who is quoting selectively? In my paper I started by discussing the WHO guidelines, where the only support came from Hu's paper (see Chapter 2) and where they had excluded thirty similar studies with contradictory results.

Adipose tissue levels tell you nothing about the intake of C12-16 so this discussion is useless.

That tissue levels of C12-16, the short saturated fatty acids, give us more reliable information than a dietary questionnaire was described in detail in my paper.

I also tried to publish a version of my paper in Läkartidningen. Here are some of the objections from the referees:

The paper is tendentious and not serious...

It is highly unlikely that the experienced researchers, who have written the dietary recommendations should have made such flawed conclusions as Ravnskov claims...

Much time is used for curious interpretations of the Seven Countries study...

I have hastily looked at Ravnskov's manuscript...His arguments are well-known and add nothing new...

Should we believe in Ravnskov or should we believe in the interpretation of science from others, including the WHO expert groups?

To answer Ravnskov it is necessary to examine all of his arguments in detail. This is not possible, neither is Läkartidningen the right place.

I should not have to mention that the referee's task is purely to evaluate the manuscript before its publication, not in the journal.

I sent my paper to British Medical Journal, but their referee objections were not much better:

The author may not be aware of a vast body of literature that convincingly supports the association between saturated fat and heart disease...

The evidence that saturated fat is harmful to health is overwhelming...

This paper provides no new arguments...

The author argues that the lowest cholesterol values ever measured in healthy people have been found in populations who live almost entirely on animal food. These populations e.g. the Masai and other African tribes have a completely different lifestyle than that of developed populations making this argument irrelevant...

This paper is an impassioned opinion rather than a balanced analysis.

This opinion piece is one-sided, but indirectly makes an important argument.

There were many more objections of the same nature. In a nine page letter I explained to the editor why I considered all of them irrelevant. She paid attention to my comments and sent my manuscript to a third referee. Curiously, although he found the paper interesting and recommended it for publication, it was finally rejected eight months after I had submitted it.

It is well documented that the peer review system is far from ideal. Whether a paper is accepted or not may be determined by irrelevant factors. Together with two renowned colleagues Richard Smith, a former editor of The British Medical Journal, studied this system and found it to be *slow, expensive, ineffective, something of a lottery, prone to bias and abuse, and hopeless at spotting errors and fraud.*[8]

A meeting at the National Heart, Lung, and Blood Institute

A workshop was organized in 1994 in Bethesda entitled Analysis of Cholesterol-Lowering Trials and sponsored by National Heart, Lung, and Blood Institute. All scientists who had published a meta-analysis of the trials were invited. They had forgotten to ask me. Petr Skrabanek and John McCormick, two British researchers who also had published an analysis with a negative outcome were not invited either. I wrote to the secretary and asked if we weren't welcome. He sent me an apology, and of course, we were most welcome. My British colleagues did not come, however. I assume that they had realized that their participation would not be likely to change anything.

I was offered ten minutes for my presentation.

I reminded the audience about the lack of association between blood cholesterol and the lack of association between blood cholesterol and the degree of atherosclerosis. I also pointed to the many studies which had shown that high cholesterol was not a risk factor and showed them the result of my meta-analysis.

I can't recall any response except that the moderator asked me inquisitorially if there wasn't anything that could convince me, and when I wanted to comment on the other presentations, I wasn't allowed to use the microphone.

Afterwards Basil Rifkind, head of the National Heart, Lung, and Blood Institute and the director of the LRC trial angrily asked me, who had sponsored my research. It was obvious that he did not believe that I had paid for everything myself. I regret that I did not ask him who had supported his research. It is not a secret that the food and drug industries regularly pay large amounts to the institute and its researchers, but it would have been interesting to hear his answer.

A meeting in Stockholm

In 1992 the Swedish National Food Administration held a course named 'Fat and Fatty Acids – Recent Scientific Findings' which was directed at dietitians and other people interested in dietary problems. Then a large number of studies had shown that there was no association between blood cholesterol and the intake of saturated fat, that heart patients had not eaten more saturated fat before they fell ill than other people, and that the dietary trials had failed in reducing the risk of heart disease. Professor Lars Werkö and myself were curious to know if the Food Administration had changed their mind and we decided to register for the course.

Apparently the lecturers had not taken any notice of the scientific news and accordingly, we asked many inquisitive questions. After some time Åke Bruce, the head of the Food Administration asked us to stop because it took too much time away from the lectures. Instead he would arrange a conference, where we could discuss the issue with other experts.

A one-day conference was held six months later in Stockholm with about forty participants from Scandinavia and the UK. Apart from Werkö, myself and two colleagues with a critical view on the dietary guidelines, all of them were well-known supporters of the cholesterol campaign. Werkö and I were given ten minutes each to present our view; the rest of the talks were given by our opponents.

Nevertheless, we succeeded in raising an animated debate after each presentation, and a summary of the talks including all comments from the audience was recorded in written form and a summary was published by the Food Administration.[9]

However, our well-founded objections had no effect whatsoever on the dietary guidelines that were updated shortly after.

Sources

1. Hecht HS, Superko HR. JACC 2001;37:1506-11.
2. Ravnskov U. J Clin Epidemiol 1995;48:713-719.
3. Olsson AG. Läkartidningen 2005;102:1393-4.
4. LaRosa JC and others. N Engl J Med 2005;352:1425-35.
5. Ravnskov U. Läkartidningen 2005;102:2593-4.
6. Olsson AG. Läkartidningen 2006;103:569
7. Ravnskov U. QJM 2002;95:397-403
8. Smith R. The Trouble with Medical Journals. 2006. The Royal Society of Medicine Press.
9. Swedish National Food Administration. Rapport 2/94.

CHAPTER 13
When Arguments Stop Working

The mama looked down and spit on the ground
Everytime my name gets mentioned
The papa said oy if I get that boy
I'm gonna stick him in the house of detention

Paul Simon

'Here logic fails – raise your voice!' These were the words of a member of the clergy, written in the margin of his Sunday prayer. And this is also a method used ocassionally when the cholesterol authorities are unable to ignore the critics.

On television
When I published my first book, 'The Cholesterol Myth', in Swedish in 1991 I was invited to appear on a Danish television program to discuss the issue with a local rabbit researcher, Børge Nordestgaard. Finally, I thought naively, now I have a chance to tell the truth to everybody.

In the studio somebody had placed a large bowl filled with giant pieces of boiled lard that quivered with the slightest touch of the table. I realized that this was not a good opening.

Nordestgaard started the discussion. He called me an outsider with strange views in conflict with a whole world of experts. To invite me to a television show was a foolish decision, because in Denmark there were many experts with much better knowledge about the subject. At the end of the program I was allowed to speak for two minutes. I had no practical knowledge about debating in public then so I assume that my words made little impact.

My book was translated into Finnish. Shortly after it was published I was contacted by Finnish television. They sent a reporter and a photographer to my home in Sweden to interview me. When the program was aired, each of my statements was followed by lengthy comments from the local Finnish experts whom I have questioned in my book, and at the end of the program my book was set on fire.

In close-up, its cover with Leonardo da Vinci's drawing of the human heart was converted into ashes.

In 2004 the Dutch medical journalist Melchior Meijer published an article about statins and their adverse effects in Algemeen Dagblad, a major Dutch newspaper. Its title was 'Statins - Miracle Drug or Tragedy?' In his article he mentioned the many potential adverse effects and the fact that their trivial benefit was independent of the degree of cholesterol lowering. He discussed the many ways that the pharmaceutical industry makes their drugs look harmless and gave a short recapitulation of Graveline's memory loss.

The article led to furious attacks on Meijer. In a primetime television show, doctors and peer journalists accused him of deliberately spreading false and potentially deadly information. He finally ended up before the Dutch Press Council, accused by a pharma-sponsored patient organization. The Council concluded however that *although the article is coloured, the author presented enough journalistic evidence to write such a piece.*

In 2007 I was contacted by TrosRadar television, a program which provides consumer news in the Netherlands. Its director had become interested in the issue after Meijer's article and its consequences. As I was the most outspoken critic of the cholesterol campaign they wanted to hear my view and sent a film team to Sweden to interview me. Meijer, a critical Dutch cardiologist, and two patients who had experienced serious side effects from their statin treatment, participated as well.

The show resulted in a media earthquake. More than 6000 people with adverse effects from statin treatment contacted TrosRadar. People from Unilever, Pfizer and the Dutch Association of Cardiology responded as well. They contacted 'De Leugen Regeert' (The lie rules), a television program which is aimed at investigating and criticizing journalists. On the show, broadcasted a week later, Martijn Katan, one of the leading cholesterol experts in The Netherlands, described me as an eccentric and irresponsible headbanger who had been kicked out of the universities in Copenhagen and Lund, a misfit whom no Danish hospital would dream of employing. A few days later he repeated his slander on the radio.

TrosRadar checked my background and when they realized that none of the many allegations were true, they aired a new TV program in which Katan was described as a liar. They offered him and my other critics an opportunity to meet me in person on a new television show, but they declined, with the excuse that they discussed such matters only with real scientists.

For several days Pfizer published large advertisements in the Dutch newspapers, where they warned people against stopping their statin treatment. Little by little the issue abated, but two of the critics, the cardiologists Martijn Katan and John Kastelein didn't forget me.

Martijn B. Katan

A strong argument against the vilification of saturated fat is Ronald Krauss' finding that the number of the 'bad', small, dense LDL particles goes down when we eat saturated fat. In 2008 Katan and his co-workers published a paper in which they presented the usual view about saturated fat and its effect on the blood lipids.[1] In a letter to the editor[2] in which I commented on Katan's paper, I reminded the authors about Krauss' findings.

Katan answered[3] that the replacement of saturated fat with other nutrients *unequivocally lowers cholesterol concentrations; all meta-analyses of controlled trials agree on this.* He added that I had published approximately 58 Letters to the editor of various medical journals. *All my letters have argued essentially the same point, namely that lowering blood cholesterol concentrations is of unproven value. I agree with the dozens of scientists who have carefully replied to his letters and who have shown that, by and large, his arguments are faulty.*

As is customary in scientific publications, the statements in my letter were followed by references to my sources, in this case to Krauss' papers. Katan only stated that all agree. Obviously he had not read my 58 'letters' himself, because his list included not only letters, but also a number of lengthy reviews and a paper about a botanical issue authored by a kin of mine. It is also easy to see that the issues of the letters, which I have published, varies considerably.

John Kastelein

In a letter published in the British Medical Journal, I mentioned the many contradictory results from studies of people with familial hypercholesterolemia.[4] I concluded that it could not possibly be the high cholesterol in these people that caused a few of them to die early from a heart attack and presented another explanation (see Chapter 3).

John Kastelein is another Dutch cholesterol expert who for many years has published 40-50 papers every year about that subject. Most of them are reports from experiments with statins on thousands of patients and healthy people. How he is able to manage that (one report each week) is a mystery.

Of course he need not waste time applying for research money because he is supported by nine different drug com-panies. Kastelein was also one of the participants who vilified me on Dutch television.

After the publication of my letter in British Medical Journal, I received an e-mail from Kastelein, who had sent copies to five of his colleagues as well. He started the letter with *Dear mister Ravnskov* and described my view on statin treatment as *criminal and bordering on the insane*. He made it clear that I was lucky not to live in the Netherlands, or else he would have dragged me to court. He asked me to read his paper about familial hypercholesterolemia in the eighteenth century (see Chapter 3) as well as his report from the JUPITER trial. According to Kastelein, *these papers completely contradicted all of my ridiculous contentions*. He ended the letter with the following statement: *Your nonsense is creating an anger in me that I have not experienced for a long time.*

Sweden

In 1997 Finnish and American researchers in cooperation had studied several thousand healthy people for a number of years. At follow-up they compared the diet of those who had suffered a heart attack during the observation period with the diet of the others. To their surprise they found that the latter group on average had not eaten more saturated fat than had the heart patients; in fact they had eaten a little less.[5] I was not surprised, because more than twenty similar studies had produced similar results, but the new study gave me the idea to present the issue in Dagens Nyheter, a major Swedish newspaper.

On the publication day a journalist from Swedish television called me and asked me to participate on the News Program. However, on my answering machine the same evening she told me that the interview had been cancelled. The reason was that she had talked with a couple of Swedish cholesterol experts who had told her that I had misunderstood the paper.

Afterwards, two of the experts used by the Swedish Food Admini-stration, published a critical paper in Läkartidningen.[6] Here they stated that the Board of the Swedish Society of Medicine had previously con-sidered creating a fire brigade of medical experts who should be on hand to clear up any blatantly indiscriminate statements, in an authoritative manner. The project was cancelled because they realized that individual actors' motives and appetite for media attention could preclude the task:

The symbiosis between a crank, eager to discuss and to boost his book, and a deputy holiday-editor was obviously irresistible. Against such a mixture Science is fighting in vain.

I hadn't mentioned my book in the article, however; it had been out of print for several years.

Spoofing

This is a technique used by clever experts in information technology. In some way they are able to send an e-mail message using another person's name as the originating sender. This method can obviously be used to harm an opponent's reputation by transmitting false and malicious e-mail communications. A women from the US sent an indignant letter to me because of an e-mail message which she thought I had sent her. The false letter opened with the words, *You really need to get a clue, you stinky buttholed woman.* After that the recipient was told to read my papers and my homepage to understand that the cholesterol campaign was a hoax. The letter was filled with insults and foul language and signed with my name. It ended with the words *You are truly a STUPID FUCK.*

I told her that I was not the sender and appreciated her for having contacted me. How many know that the name which appears as the sender of an e-mail message is not necessarily the person who has sent the message? I also wonder how many people have received that particular letter?

Sources

1. Katan MB. Am J Clin Nutr 2006;83:989–90
2. Ravnskov U. Am J Clin Nutr 2006;84:1550-1
3. www.proteinpower.com/drmike/lipid-hypothesis/saturated-fat-debate
4. www.bmj.com/cgi/eletters/337/aug27_2/a1095#202758
   Ravnskov U. BMJ 2008;337:a1681
5. Pietinen P and others. Am J Epidemiol 1997;145:876-87.
6. Becker W, Rössner S. Läkartidningen 1997;94:4259-60.

CHAPTER 14
Industrial Tricks

Everybody! Oh Lord, won't you buy me a Mercedes Benz?
My friends all drive Porsches, I must make amends,
Worked hard all my lifetime, no help from my friends,
So oh Lord, won't you buy me a Mercedes Benz?

Janis Joplin

Most of what I tell you about in this chapter is taken from two important books written by people with inside information. The first one is 'The Truth About The Drug Companies' by Marcia Angell, former editor-in-chief of the New England Journal of Medicine, one of the world's largest and most respected medical journals. The other one is 'The Trouble With Medical Journals' by Richard Smith, former editor-in-chief of the British Medical Journal, another great and respectable publication.

I have included only a few examples of the ways in which we are misled. Anyone who still thinks that medical science is an independent enterprise, aimed at discovering the causes of our diseases and the best way to prevent or treat them, is urged to read these books from cover to cover.

A drug trial is extremely costly and laborious. The only one willing to spend several hundred million dollars on a clinical trial is the producer of the drug and they do it because the potential profit is gigantic, in particular for producers of drugs aimed at treating healthy people for the reset of their life. Consider for example, that in 2002 the combined profits for the ten drug companies on the global business magazine Fortune's 500 list were greater than the profits for all the other 490 businesses put together. Another impressive piece of information is that in the same year the estimated sales for prescription drugs worldwide was about $400 billion, a figure that is even higher today.

Before 1980 researchers who wanted to test a new drug received a grant from its producer, but the latter had no influence whatsoever on the way the trial was run. Thanks to new legislation the situation has changed radically.

Today the drug companies pay for the necessary meetings, workshops, conferences, fees for speakers and authors and travel expenses for hundreds of participating doctors and researchers in each trial. They prepare the trials, take part in the selection of patients and the control group individuals, specify the study design and produce the protocols, participate in monitoring the results and the analysis of blood cholesterol. They are also responsible for the complicated statistical calculations and they decide whether a clinical trial report shall be published or not, at least they did until a few years ago.

Even the trial reports are in the hands of Big Pharma. In many cases PR firms write them and when completed, the drug company asks renowned researchers to put their name on the top. According to Richard Smith many medical journals are packed with articles ghostwritten by pharmaceutical companies, but their influence goes further. Listen for instance to Marcia Angell:

Researchers serve as consultants to companies whose products they are studying, become paid members of advisory boards and speakers bureaus, enter into patent and royalty arrangements together with their institutions, promote drugs and devices at company-sponsored symposiums, and allow themselves to be plied with expensive gifts and trips to luxurious settings, and many also have equity interest in the companies.

Even the most prestigious universities are supported generously. For instance, Harvard Medical School is sponsored by a dozen of the major drug companies. BigPharma has also invaded the National Institutes of Health, where all the governmental research grants and funding are administered. A large number of senior scientists supplement their already high income by accepting large consulting fees and stock options from drug companies that have dealings with their institutions.

The practising doctors have lucrative financial arrangements with BigPharma as well. For instance, in the US they are paid more than $10,000 for each patient they enroll in a drug trial, and after the sixth patient they can expect a further $30,000.

How is all that possible and is it legal? It is legal because the drug industry's long arm reaches into legislation. The pharmaceutical industry has by far the largest lobby in Washington. In 2002 the number was 675 lobbyists, more than one for each member of Congress. They also know how to exert an influence because 26 of these lobbyists were former Congress members and 342 had been otherwise connected with government officials. BigPharma's influence reaches higher up, however.

For example, the former Defence Secretary Donald Rumsfield was chief executive officer, president and the chairman of Searle, a major drug firm, now owned by Pfizer. Mitchell E.Daniels jr., former White House budget director, was senior vice president of Eli Lilly, and the first President Bush was on the Eli Lilly board of directors before becoming president. As Marcia Angell commented, *The connections are so close that annual meetings of PhRMA look like Washington power conclaves.*

What is PhRMA You may ask. Most US drug companies are organized in the Pharmaceutical Research and Manufacturers of America, or PhRMA. According to its homepage, this organization claims to be *the country's leading pharmaceutical research and biotechnology companies, which are devoted to inventing medicines that allow patients to live longer, healthier, and more productive lives. PhRMA companies are leading the way in the search for new cures.*

If you exchange the word 'patients' with 'doctors and scientists, drug company employees and stockholders,' you are probably somewhat closer to the truth.

The guideline authors

Guidelines for preventing 'the great killer' cardiovascular disease are supposed to be written by impartial scientists. At least we expect that if any of their authors have financial connections to a drug company, the reader should be informed. When the guidelines from the National Cholesterol Education Program were published in the medical journal Circulation in 2004, no financial disclosures were given. After a letter from Merrill Goozner of the Center for Science in the Public Interest who questioned the scientific basis and objectivity of the guidelines, the financial disclosures were published on the web, but not in the journal, where the guidelines had been published. Here they are:

Dr. Grundy *has received honoraria from Merck, Pfizer, Sankyo, Bayer, Merck/ Schering-Plough, Kos, Abbott, Bristol-Myers Squibb, and AstraZeneca; he has received research grants from Merck, Abbott, and Glaxo Smith Kline.*

Dr. Cleeman *has no financial relationships to disclose.*

Dr. Bairey Merz *has received lecture honoraria from Pfizer, Merck, and Kos; she has served as a consultant for Pfizer, Bayer, and EHC (Merck); she has received unrestricted institutional grants for Continuing Medical Education from Pfizer, Procter & Gamble, Novartis, Wyeth, AstraZeneca, and Bristol-Myers Squibb Medical Imaging.*

She has received a research grant from Merck; she has stock in Boston Scientific, IVAX, Eli Lilly, Medtronic, Johnson & Johnson, SCIPIE Insurance, ATS Medical, and Biosite.

Dr. Brewer *has received honoraria from AstraZeneca, Pfizer, Lipid Sciences, Merck, Merck/Schering-Plough, Fournier, Tularik, Esperion, and Novartis; he has served as a consultant for AstraZeneca, Pfizer, Lipid Sciences, Merck, Fournier, Tularik, Sankyo, Merck/Schering-Plough, and Novartis.*

Dr. Clark *has received honoraria for educational presentations from Abbott, AstraZeneca, Bristol-Myers Squibb, Merck, and Pfizer; he has received grant/research support from Abbott, AstraZeneca, Bristol-Myers Squibb, Merck, and Pfizer.*

Dr. Hunninghake *has received honoraria for consulting and speakers bureau from AstraZeneca, Merck, Merck/Schering-Plough, and Pfizer, and for consulting from Kos; he has received research grants from AstraZeneca, Bristol-Myers Squibb, Kos, Merck, Merck/Schering-Plough, Novartis, and Pfizer.*

Dr. Pasternak *has served as a speaker for Pfizer, Merck, Merck/Schering-Plough, Takeda, Kos, BMS-Sanofi, and Novartis; he has served as a consultant for Merck, Merck/Schering-Plough, Sanofi, Pfizer Health Solutions, Johnson & Johnson Merck, and AstraZeneca.*

Dr. Smith *has received institutional research support from Merck; he has stocks in Medtronic and Johnson & Johnson.*

Dr. Stone *has received honoraria for educational lectures from Abbott, Astra-Zeneca, Bristol-Myers Squibb, Kos, Merck, Merck/Schering-Plough, Novartis, Pfizer, Reliant, and Sankyo; he has served as a consultant for Abbott, Merck, Merck/Schering-Plough, Pfizer, and Reliant.*

More tricks

According to an FBI press release on September 2, 2009, Pfizer published the results of a Valdecoxib (Bextra®) trial in a manner that obscured the risks and pleaded guilty to numerous charges of false advertisements. Pfizer agreed to pay $2.3 billion, which is the largest health care fraud settlement in the history of the Department of Justice; the largest criminal fine of any kind imposed in the US and the largest ever civil fraud settlement against a pharmaceutical company.

In Chapter 3 I told you about the ENHANCE trial. In this trial Merck and Schering-Plough tested their new non-statin drug ezetimibe together with simvastatin and found that the result in the ezetimibe group was worse than in the simvastatin group.

Although this was known shortly after the termination of the trial, they did not tell anybody about it until two years later. During that time sales of Vytorin generated billions of dollars in annual sales.

And there is more. On September 30, 2004, Merck withdrew their painkiller rofecoxib (Vioxx®), another multibillion dollar drug. The reason? It was good at relieving pain, but at the same time many of its users died from a heart attack. At the FDA, they had estimated that in the five years the drug was on the market, Vioxx had caused more than 100,000 heart attacks in the US, a third of which were fatal. Afterwards, it appeared that Merck had been aware of the risk for four years.

As a part of the process the court got access to Merck's archives and found that most articles about Vioxx were prepared by Merck's own scientists or by medical publishing companies. For example, seventy-two reviews were published between 1999 and 2003, but only a few had actually been written by those who were named as authors. Instead, Merck had hired outside firms to write drafts, which were then sent to the prominent scientists. They were asked to review the manuscripts before they put their name at the top and got paid. When the papers were published, half of them did not mention the name of the real author, neither did they mention the names of the sponsors.

The manipulation is disgusting. I just didn't realize the extent, said Catherine DeAngelis, editor-in-chief of The Journal of The American Medical Association, to CNN.

Fake journals

Elsevier is the world's largest publisher of medical and scientific literature. It is the owner of more than 2000 journals and several major publishing companies, among which are Academic Press, Churchill Livingstone, Excerpta Medica, Pergamon Press and Saunders. During the Vioxx scandal it appeared that Merck had paid Elsevier for publishing six Australian medical journals that at first glance had looked like peer-reviewed journals, but the journals had contained only articles favourable to drugs produced by Merck, while the articles were ghostwritten by writers who had been paid by the drug company.

More problems

Most medical journals are unable to survive without their income from the drug companies, and financial conflicts of interest are therefore ubiquitous. Papers that report favourable effects of new drugs are used to market the drug to doctors in many countries.

To do that its producer orders huge numbers of reprints of the report. If an editor rejects the report because it is considered of inferior quality, the journal may lose more than a million dollars from reprint sales.

A major source of income is advertisements, most of which come from the drug industry, and if editors accept a paper which is too critical of the pharmaceutical industry or their products, they put the survival of the journal at risk. For example, when a study about misleading pharmaceutical advertising was published in Annals of Internal Medicine, it resulted in a severe drop in advertising income and the premature departure of their editors. The journal survived because it is one of the largest and most influential ones; smaller journals might have ended their life. The owners know that this is a likely outcome, as do the editors.

Marcia Angell is merciless in her conclusions: *All of this makes a mockery of the traditional role of researchers as independent and impartial scientists.*

Part Three

CHAPTER 15
The Real Cause?

The mind is like a parachute - it works only when it is open

Frank Zappa

To suppress or distort information in science may produce many unfortunate consequences. Huge amounts of money and personnel are wasted in the pursuit of blind paths, millions of healthy people are converted into patients and perhaps worse of all, new, more fecund ideas are suppressed, either by the inventors themselves or by their colleagues.

Progress in science depends mainly or entirely on disagreement, but if new ideas that go contrary to established 'knowledge' are considered as a sign of ignorance or stupidity, nothing happens. Nevertheless, let me, against all odds, present a hypothesis that is able to explain the many observations that are now impossible to fit in with current wisdom. I have explained it in my previous book, 'Fat and Cholesterol Are GOOD for You!' Because it may be somewhat difficult to understand, for people without knowledge about human anatomy and pathology, I shall try to do it again in another way. You can find a more scientific explanation and more references in a paper that I published recently together with my colleague Kilmer McCully.[1]

Infection and inflammation

Most likely there are many causes of coronary heart disease, and some of them we know for certain. There is no doubt that smoking, diabetes and mental stress may provoke a heart attack. What we do not know is the mechanism. How come that different causes may lead to the same disease? We think we know the answer, but please remember that our explanation is a hypothesis. We may be wrong, and those who have lived in the cholesterol world for many years will probably shake their head in disbelief.

The first part of our hypothesis is not our own. It was proposed more than hundred years ago and it says, to express it very simply, that atherosclerosis is the result of an infection in the arterial wall.

The second part explains why and how LDL-cholesterol and the microorganisms end up here and what happens before a thrombus is created inside the artery.

Most researchers agree that atherosclerosis starts as an inflammation in the arterial wall. There is also a general agreement that atherosclerosis, heart disease and stroke are associated in some way with infectious diseases. For example, remnants from more than fifty different bacterial species[2] and a number of viruses as well[3] have been identified in atherosclerotic tissue, and antibodies against several of these microorganisms are present in abnormally high amounts in the blood of patients with cardiovascular disease and in people who die from it later in life.

One hundred years ago many researchers considered atherosclerosis as an infectious disease. It was known that people who died from an infection were more atherosclerotic if they had been infected a long time before death than if they had acquired the infection a few days before.[4] The following statement by two American pathologists, Oskar Klotz and M. F. Manning is typical for the general view at that time: *There is every indication that the production of tissue in the intima (the innermost layer of the arterial wall) is the result of a direct irritation of that tissue by the presence of infection or toxins.*[5]

Today more than one hundred reviews about this issue have been published in medical journals. However, almost all authors appear to think that the infections are secondary; that the microorganisms locate to atherosclerotic tissue because here they are able to multiply without being disturbed by our immune system.

What most researchers also accept is that the starting point of an occluding thrombus is a soft bubble lying just beneath the inner surface of the artery wall. It is called a vulnerable plaque, discovered by Danish pathologist Erling Falk. He examined the hearts of patients who had died because of an acute myocardial infarction and noted that the occluding thrombus usually was situated close to a ruptured bubble.[6]

Now to the crucial questions. What is causing the inflammation and how is the vulnerable plaque created?

According to the present view the first step is what researchers call activation of the arterial endothelium, the thin cell layer that cover the inside of all vessels. There are many factors that are said to activate or irritate the endothelium, for instance the toxic chemicals present in tobacco smoke, too little vitamins or copper in our food, and too much iron or homocysteine in our blood.

Homocysteine is an amino acid normally present in minute amounts. If its concentration is too high the risk of cardiovascular disease increases. Children born with an extremely high level of homocysteine due to an inborn error of metabolism rapidly become atherosclerotic and may die before the age of ten from a stroke or a heart attack.

Some researchers think that microbes circulating in the blood may attack the endothelium, in particular if it has been damaged by toxic factors, but the prevailing idea is that high LDL cholesterol is the main culprit. When the endothelium is made active, a condition named endothelial dysfunction, it is said to allow LDL-cholesterol to pass through the endothelial cells and enter the intima, the innermost layer of the arterial wall.

That LDL-cholesterol enter the intima when it is activated is also a hypothesis. It is a necessary assumption to explain why so much cholesterol is found in the arterial wall, because normally, cholesterol is not able to enter an endothelial cell or any other cell for that matter. The activated endothelium is also said to attract a type of white blood cells named monocytes and invite them to enter the interior of the arterial wall.

When LDL-cholesterol has passed through the endothelial cells, they are said to be attacked by cells in the intima resulting in a change of their structure; LDL becomes oxidized. It is this process which is considered as the cause of inflammation. After having been oxidized the monocytes, now converted to macrophages, take up the oxidized LDL-cholesterol.

I have not yet found anyone who has been able to tell me why LDL molecules become oxidized, just because they enter the arterial wall, but this is the official explanation, which is necessary to explain the next step.

The foam cell
Now it is time to introduce the foam cell, an important actor in the process of atherosclerosis. The foam cell is a type of white blood cell called a macrophage, but it doesn't look like a normal macrophage. It's interior is filled with small bubbles that give the viewer the impression that it is loaded with foam. It isn't foam, however, it is lipid droplets.

Like many other white blood cells macrophages are able to take up foreign material, such as bacteria and viruses, but also normal molecules that have been damaged, like oxidized LDL molecules. At least it is said so, because it is a necessary assumption to be able to explain how foam cells are created.

Foam cells mount up in rows just beneath the endothelial cells and are visible with the naked eye as yellowish stripes on the inside of the larger arteries. In the surrounding tissue outside the cells there are also many lipid droplets. The usual interpretation is that these droplets represent oxidized LDL cholesterol, identical with those seen inside the macrophages.

All people, even foetuses, have fatty streaks in varying amounts, and their number increases after birth. Later in childhood fewer are seen, but their number increases again in young adults. Elderly people have few fatty streaks, but more atherosclerotic plaques.[7]

Fatty streaks are considered as an early stage of atherosclerosis because they are often seen at the same places in the arteries where the atherosclerotic plaques usually are situated later in life. However, that small children have fewer fatty streaks than newborns tells us that they also may be temporary. We think that fatty streaks is a normal and harmless phenomenon. The question is, whether some of them turn into atherosclerotic plaques, and why.

It is necessary to assume that the LDL molecules in the droplets are oxidized before they are taken up by the macrophages because like other cells, the macrophages do not take up normal LDL molecules. As you may remember from the Nobel Prize chapter, uptake of cholesterol demands that the cholesterol door, the LDL receptor, is open, and it doesn't open unless the cell needs extra cholesterol. The macrophage is said to have a backdoor, however, through which foreign guests, for instance oxidized LDL, can enter.

Another possibility, which we consider more likely, is that the droplets are taken up by phagocytosis. This is the way in which white blood cells engulf and destroy microorganisms and for a special reason it may work in this way with the lipid droplets as well. I shall soon tell you why.

The contradictions

The mechanism I have described above is in conflict with most of what has been observed in this field of medical science. I have mentioned most of the contradictions previously, but it is worthwhile to do it repeatedly and again.

Why do people with low cholesterol become just as atherosclerotic as people with high cholesterol?

Why do people with high cholesterol live the longest?

Why is high cholesterol not a risk factor for women?

Why is the degree of endothelial dysfunction the same in people with high cholesterol as in people with low?[8]

Why do normal cells oxidize normal LDL molecules?

Endothelial dysfunction is pronounced in atherosclerotic children who are born with excessive amounts of homocysteine in the blood, so-called hyperhomocysteinuria. Why isn't there any cholesterol present in their arteries.[9]

Furthermore, no one has explained how the dangerous bubbles, which Falk found in the artery walls, are created. Therefore, let me describe them in more detail.

The vulnerable plaque

In the microscope the interior of the bubble is a mess of dead tissue containing many red and white blood cells, cholesterol crystals and lipid droplets looking just like those lying inside the foam cells. In the microscope the vulnerable plaques look like bubbles in the endothelium, only separated from the interior of the arteries by a thin membrane. They can be seen in other arteries as well, for instance in the carotid arteries, those that transport blood to the brain. By use of a catheter pushed into the arteries and provided with a thermometer in the tip, it has been shown that their temperature is a little higher than that of the surrounding tissue.[10]

Another interesting finding is the numerous lipid droplets that are found in the inflamed arterial wall outside the vulnerable plaques. They are rarely seen directly beneath the endothelium like the foam cells, as should be expected if LDL cholesterol entered by way of the endothelium, but much deeper.[11] This observation is crucial for the understanding of our hypothesis. Before I go into more detail it is necessary to tell you more about the lipoproteins. Most researchers today think that their main function is to carry cholesterol, but they have also other important functions.

The lipoprotein immune system

Sixty years ago researchers discovered that the lipoproteins participate in our immune system by binding and inactivating bacteria, viruses and their toxic products.[1] The lipoprotein immune system may be particularly important in early childhood, because in contrast to the antibody-producing system, which needs repeated stimulations to function properly, the lipoproteins work immediately and with great efficiency. There are many ways to demonstrate it.

One example is that researchers have looked at mixtures of lipoproteins and bacterial toxins with an electron microscope. What they saw was that the toxin molecules stuck to each other and became attached to the LDL molecules,[12] and similar experiments with virus gave the same result.[13]

In the laboratory it has been shown that human LDL is able to inactivate more than 90% of the most toxic bacterial products.[14] When Kenneth Feingold and his co-workers at the University of California in San Francisco reduced blood cholesterol in rats and gave them an injection of bacterial toxin, most of them died quickly but if they injected a purified human LDL beforehand, they survived.[15] Mihai Netea and his team from the University Hospital in Nijmegen found that this is not necessary if they used mice with familial hypercholesterolemia. Most of such mice survived, whereas normal mice died immediately, a beautiful proof that high cholesterol is advantageous.[16]

When we are attacked by microbes, the white blood cells send a message to the liver by excreting their hormones, the cytokines. The liver responds by increasing the production of lipoprotein including the 'bad' LDL; yet another indication that LDL is a useful molecule. Most surprising is that apart from those who have been directly involved in the research in this field, very few know anything about this system, not even experts in infectious diseases or immunology, and hitherto I have not found a word about it in any current textbook.

The new hypothesis

When the lipoproteins bind the toxic intruders to their surface, all of them, toxins, microorganisms and lipoproteins, aggregate, meaning that they lump together into microscopic clumps that circulate in the blood. One contributing factor may be the anti-oxLDL-antibodies. Antibodies have two arms and are therefore able to bind two oxidized LDL-particles at the same time. Also, if too much homocysteine is present in the blood, it reacts with LDL molecules and makes them lump together.

In our view these particles play a crucial role in the creation of the vulnerable plaque. I shall soon explain in which way, but first a question: What is a vulnerable plaque? Doesn't it look like something all of us know very well?

Probably you have already guessed it, but here is what we think: the vulnerable plaque is a pustule, a small boil.

Its interior looks like the interior of a boil, its temperature is higher than the surrounding tissue, just as is the case with a boil, and it may burst and empty its content like a boil.

Boils and pustules are characterized by a special type of white blood cells called neutrophil granulocytes. In the inflamed atherosclerotic tissue some other types dominate, the so-called B and T-cells, those that belong to the antibody-producing system. Neutrophil granulocytes are rare except in the region around the vulnerable plaques,[17] a further indication that it is a pustule.

Pustules are created by microorganisms. If the vulnerable plaque is a pustule, it should contain the responsible microorganisms as well, and when it bursts, they should enter the arterial blood and create symptoms similar to any other infectious disease. Indeed, patients with an acute heart attack often have fever, chills and some sweating. They also have leucocytosis (too many white blood cells in the blood), and high levels of the same blood constituents that are elevated in infections, for instance CRP, and in about a fifth of patients with cardiogenic shock (life-threatening heart attacks) living bacteria are present in the blood.[18] It is also in accordance with our hypothesis that large numbers of neutrophil granulocytes are found almost always in the heart tissue about 24 hours after an acute heart attack.

The idea is not new. As far as we know it was first suggested by Sir William Osler, the Canadian pathologist and physician who became the Regius Professor of Medicine at Oxford and a leading physician of his time. In one of his papers he described the vulnerable plaque as *an atherosclerotic pustule*.[19]

But how is the boil created? Here is our explanation.

The mechanism

When the blood is pumped into the tissues by the heart it goes through a complicated mesh of vessels. The first one, the largest artery in the body, is the aorta. All organs in the body (other than the lungs), including the heart and the brain, are supplied by branches from the aorta. When an artery enters an organ it splits up into smaller arteries named arterioles and each arteriole splits up into capillaries, the smallest vessels in the body, visible only with a microscope. The width of a capillary is so small that it forces red blood cells to fold to be able to pass through. The capillaries supply the tissues with oxygen and nutrients and after that they join as venules and veins that return the blood to the heart, from where it is pumped to the lungs.

Even the walls of the larger vessels such as arteries and veins are nourished through capillaries, the so-called vasa vasorum, which surround these vessels like an intricate meshwork.

What we suggest is that the LDL clumps may become so numerous and of a size that they are able to obstruct the vasa vasorum. Consequently small parts of the arterial walls become malnourished, get too little oxygen and may even die. You could say that they cause a small infarct of the artery wall. The toxic passengers of the obstructing clumps may now escape from the LDL prison and start multiplying in the dead tissue, which therefore becomes inflamed.

That too little oxygen is available, a condition named hypoxia, has been shown by intricate chemical analysis of atherosclerotic arteries. Hypoxia is most pronounced in the deeper parts of the inflamed arterial walls where the macrophages are dominant.[20]

If the immune system is OK, the surrounding white blood cells and the antibodies attack the microorganisms. Fibroblasts and new capillaries grow into the inflamed tissue and eventually it will be transformed into a scar, the fibrous plaque. If not, a pustule is created, its thin membrane may burst, the content of the plaque flows out into the blood, a clot is created at the margins and if it becomes too large the blood flow become obstructed and the tissue that is nourished by the artery dies. If it happens in a coronary artery the result is a heart attack; if it happens in a carotid artery the result is a stroke; if it happens in an artery that goes to the eye, the victim may become partially blind.

Everything fits

There is much evidence supporting the idea that inflammation of the arteries is not the primary cause of heart attacks or strokes, but a secondary phenomenon caused by the microorganisms or their toxins. They are not settling in the atherosclerotic plaques because they are safe there; vulnerable plaques may occur anywhere, also in normal arteries, which explains why a heart attack may be seen also in people with completely normal arteries.

The primary cause is not the microbes either; it is the factors which stimulate their growth or make our immune system fail. It is not the water that causes the boat to go down; it is the iceberg that has staved in the keel.

That the microbes play an important role is obvious, and the evidence is right before our noses. For instance, mortality in myocardial infarction and stroke increases during influenza epidemics[21] and people with infected teeth[22] or with bacteria in the blood[22] are at greater risk than healthy people.

Furthermore, about one-third of all patients with acute myocardial infarction or stroke have had an infectious disease immediately before onset.[24] All kinds of infectious diseases may be responsible. Most common are respiratory diseases, but other types have been described as well, such as tuberculosis, HIV, tooth and urinary tract infections.

If a vulnerable plaque may appear in normal arteries, and if microorganisms cause stroke and myocardial infarction, then vascular disease may occur in all ages. This is true also. Finnish researcher Erkki Pesonen and his team noted that the coronary arteries were narrowed in children with infectious diseases, both in those who died and those who survived.[25] Stroke may even appear in early childhood, and a Canadian research team found that about a third of these children suffered from chickenpox a few months before.[26]

If inflammation was primary, anti-inflammatory drugs should be of benefit, but they are not. On the contrary, the Vioxx-scandal told us that such treatment increases the risk of heart disease, and other anti-inflammatory drugs have the same effect.[27]

Skeptics may object that statin treatment is of benefit and statins are anti-inflammatory. This is correct, but statins have many other effects; e.g. they inhibit the coagulation of the blood by enhancing a process called fibrinolysis and by slowing down the function of the blood platelets, and the platelets are necessary for the formation of blood clots. Statins are also known to stimulate the production of nitric oxide (NO), and nitric oxide makes the arteries widen. The statins would probably have a much better effect if they didn't lower cholesterol and if they weren't anti-inflammatory, because inflammation is a necessary step for normal healing of infectious processes.

Why is atherosclerosis seen only in arteries, you may ask. Veins are also supplied by vasa vasorum. Why don't the LDL-complexes obstruct the vasa vasorum of the veins? Good question, but there is a good answer also. The pressure in veins is very low, lower than in their vasa vasorum. Venous blood flows slowly and steadily and therefore, the LDL clumps have no problem passing by. In the arteries the pressure is high, much higher than in their vasa vasorum. Each stroke of the heart stops the blood flow completely in these vasa vasorum; the blood is only able to pass by during the short time when the heart is relaxed.

By the same reasoning, atherosclerotic plaques are localized to areas of the intimal surface where the hydrodynamic forces, turbulence of blood flow, and tissue pressure are especially high. This is at the branching points of the arteries and within tortuous arteries.

That atherosclerosis is seen in arteries only also contradicts the idea that microbes attack the endothelium directly. If this were true, atherosclerosis would be just as, or more common in veins.

Two other good questions are: Why is LDL oxidized in the arterial wall and how do you explain the presence of oxidized LDL?

There is a logical answer to this question. LDL is not oxidized in the arterial wall, of course. Why should our own cells attack a normal and perfect molecule with many important functions? No, LDL is oxidized after having been taken up by the macrophages together with its toxic passengers as part of a normal physiological process. When white blood cells take up foreign, dangerous material they neutralize it by oxidation and at the same time LDL is oxidized as well. Probably HDL reconstructs LDL, because laboratory experiments have shown that HDL is able to convert oxidized LDL back to normal.[28]

What about the foam cell? Is it really true that the droplets are identical with microorganisms or their toxic products captured by LDL? Have you any evidence?

Certainly! In laboratory experiments researchers have added various types of bacteria to solutions containing macrophages and human LDL. When they looked at the mixture with a microscope they saw that the previously normal macrophages had been converted to foam cells.[29] The same was observed in an experiment, where LDL was mixed with homocysteine instead of bacteria.[30]

It has been suggested that oxidized LDL cholesterol is the very cause of atherosclerosis. If so, prevention with anti-oxidative drugs should be able to prevent it, but hitherto no such experiments have been successful.

A contradiction to our hypothesis is that prevention of cardiovascular disease by antibiotics has been largely unsuccessful. However, in these experiments patients have received a single antibiotic, chosen because it was effective against a bacterium called Chlamydia pneumoniae, and the treatment was given for short periods. It is highly unlikely that such treatment should have had an effect in more than a few patients because as previously mentioned, fifty different bacteria have been localized in atherosclerotic tissue, and it is not possible to combat a virus with an antibiotic.

Prevention with antibiotics may even have the opposite effect because it may lead to the development of resistant microorganisms. It is probably a much better idea to look after bacteria in the blood in patients with an acute heart attack, and if present treat the patient with an appropriate antibiotic.

Another really useful idea is to eliminate chronic infections. Dental researchers from Italy for instance treated 35 otherwise healthy individuals with evidence of periodontal infections. After the treatment, examination of the carotid arterial wall showed that its thickness had diminished significantly and much more than seen in any cholesterol-lowering trial.[31]

Atherosclerosis is a spotty disease
According to the current ideas about atherosclerosis it should be a generalized disease. If LDL-cholesterol enters just because there is too much of it, all of our arteries should be atherosclerotic. To explain its spotty appearance it is said that atherosclerosis only occurs where the dynamic forces are especially strong, but everyone who has looked at the inside of dead people's arteries know that this is only partially true. Atherosclerosis is often located haphazardly, particularly in the aorta. This is also what we should expect if atherosclerosis was due to the effect of microbial attacks repeated again and again through our life.

The foam cells once again
We think that the presence of foam cells is a normal phenomenon. Their content may probably escape when the tissue becomes malnourished or die but most likely the lipid droplets are taken up by other macrophages, which move back into the circulation. On their way they may temporarily accumulate beneath the endothelium where they are organized as fatty streaks due to the rapid blood flow at the outside.

Foam cells are also present in other arteries, and if there are foam cells, there should be vulnerable plaques as well. They have indeed been found located to the carotids, those that carry blood to the brain.[32] Foam cells are seen beneath the retina, increasingly with advancing age.[33] They are found commonly in the glomeruli,[34] the kidneys' capillary mesh where the blood is filtered to produce urine, in particular in sclerotic glomeruli. That a glomerulus is sclerotic means that it is dead and may be compared with a scar or a fibrotic plaque. The number of sclerotic glomeruli also increases with age.

What about the risk factors?

Now to the icebergs. What do they look like and why do they stave in our boat? For many years we have been presented with a long list of risk factors for cardiovascular disease. Most of them are, with all certainty, secondary to the real cause but we think that some of them are primary, because they fit so well with our hypothesis.

Diabetes and smoking for instance are strong risk factors for all kinds of cardiovascular diseases and both diabetic patients and smokers are also susceptible to infections. Mental stress, another established risk factor, stimulates production of the hormone cortisol, and an excess of cortisol promotes infections. This is seen in patients with Cushing's disease of the adrenal glands and when cortisol is used as a treatment.

Too much homocysteine in the blood promotes the tendency for LDL to stick together. When their structure has been changed, they stimulate the immune system to produce anti-LDL-anti-bodies just as we saw in the case with oxidized LDL. Hyperhomocysteinemia is also associated with lack of vitamin B, smoking, high blood pressure, mental stress and kidney failure, and all of these conditions are risk factors for cardiovascular disease.

A final comment

If you have had the patience to read the whole book and if your cholesterol is high, I am confident that you will not bother about it any longer. You will also be able to enjoy good old-fashioned food with as much butter, cheese and cream as you choose.

But how should we avoid a heart attack or a stroke? The best way is probably to avoid what stimulates microbial growth and what is harmful to our immune system. A few suggestions are available.

There is increasing evidence that vitamin D play an important role in our immune system as a protective factor against microorganisms.[34] In accordance, a low concentration in the blood of that vitamin is also a risk factor for cardiovascular disease. Although no clinical trial have been performed to see if a supplementation with vitamin D is able to protect us, it may be a good idea to take at least 1000 IU daily, in particular during wintertime.

Our need for vitamin C is also much greater than we have been told for may years. The reason is that the amount of that vitamin inside the white blood cells is 80 times higher than in the blood.

Furthermore, glucose and vitamin C use the same cell door, meaning that if the glucose concentration is too high in the blood, these two molecules compete for access.[36] This may be why diabetics are more susceptible to infections than other people. It also means that the 50-100 mg we have been recommended as a daily amount may be far too little. One gram a day is probably a minimum for optimal health, more in case we become infected.

To learn how we can protect ourselves against microorganisms in the best way should be a challenge for curious and open-minded researchers.

Sources

1. Ravnskov U, McCully KM. Ann Clin Lab Sci 2009;39:3-16. A short version in Swedish is available in Medicinsk Access 2009;2:15-8.
2. Ott SJ and others. Circulation 2006;113:929-37.
3. Melnick JL and others. Lancet 1983;2:644-7.
   Pampou Syu and others. Virchows Arch 436, 539-52, 2000.
   Shi Y and othhers. Pathol Int 2002;52:31-9.
4. Wiesel J. Zeitschr Heilkunde 1906;27:262-94.
5. Klotz O, Manning MF. J Pathol Bacteriol 1911;16:211-20.
6. Falk E. Br Heart J 1983;50:127-34.
7. Stary HC. Atherosclerosis 61987;4:91-108.
   Stary HC. Arteriosclerosis1989;9(Suppl 1):119-32.
8. Reis SE and others. Am Heart J 2001;141:735-41.
9. McCully KM. Am J Pathol 1969;56:111-28.
   McCully KM. Clin Chem Lab Med 2005;43:980-6.
10. Madjid M and others. Am J Cardiol 2002;90(10C):36L-39L.
11. Guyton JR, Klemp KF. Am J Pathol 1993;143:1444-57
12. Bhakdi S and others. J Biol Chem 1983;258:5899-904.
13. Huemer HP and others. Intervirology 1988;29:68-76.
    Superti F and others. Med Microbiol Immunol 1992;181:77-86.
14. Flegel WA and others. Infect Immun 1989;57:2237-45.
    Cavaillon JM and others. Infect Immun 1990;58:2375-82.
    Northoff H and others. Beitr Infusionsther 1992;30:195-7.
    Flegel WA and others. Infect Immun 1993;61:5140-6.
15. Feingold KR and others. Infect Immun 1995;63:2041-6.
16. Netea MG and others. J Clin Invest 1996;97:1366-72.
17. Naruko K and others. Circulation 2002;106:2894-900.
18. Kohsaka S and others. Arch Intern Med 2005;165:1643-50.
19. Osler W. Modern Medicine: its practice and theory. Lea and Fibiger, 1908, p 426-47.
20. Sluimer JC and others. J Am Coll Cardiol 2008;51:1258-63.
21. Madjid M and others- Eur Heart J 2007;28:1205-10.
22. Spahr A and others. Arch Intrern Med 2006;166:554-9
23. Valtonen V and others. Eur Heart J 1993;14 (Suppl K): 20-3.
24. Smeeth L and others. N Engl J Med 2004;351:2611-8.

25. Pesonen E. Eur Heart J 1994;15,suppl C:57-61.
    Liuba P and others. Eur Heart J 2003;24:515-24.
26. Johnsen SP and others.Arch Intern Med 2005;165:978-84.
27. Bonnefont D and others. Clin Chem Lab Med 1999;37:939-48.
28. Kalayoglu MV and others. J Infect Dis 2000;181(Suppl 3:S483-9.
29. Qi M and others. Microb Pathog 2003;35:259-67.
30. Yuan C and others. Radiology 2001;221:285-99.
31. Piconi S and others. FASEB J 2009;23:1196-204.
32. Curcio CA and others. Invest Ophthalm Vis Sci 2001;42:265-74.
33. Schonholzer KW and others. Nephron 1992;62:130-6.
    Lee HS, Kruth HS. Nephrology 2003;8:224-30.
34. Yamshchikov AV and others. Endocrine Practice 2009;15:438-49.
    Gombart AF. Future Microbiol 2009;4:
35. Nemerovski CW and others. Pharmacotherapy 2009;29:691-708
    Judd SE and others. Am J Med Sci 2009;338:40-44.
36. Ottoboni F, Ottoboni A. J Orthomol Med 2005;20:179-83.

Acknowledgement

I am indebted to Jeff Cable for his invaluable assistance in proof-reading and in the technical preparation of the book for publishing

Index